PERFECT BONES

PERFECT BONES

A Six-Point Plan for Healthy Bones

Pamela Levin, R.N.

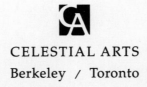

CELESTIAL ARTS

Berkeley / Toronto

Celestial Arts
P.O. Box 7123
Berkeley, California 94707
www.tenspeed.com

Distributed in Australia by Simon & Schuster Australia, in Canada by Ten Speed Press Canada, in New Zealand by Southern Publishers Group, in South Africa by Real Books, in Southeast Asia by Berkeley Books, and in the United Kingdom and Europe by Airlift Book Company.

Technical editing by Corey Cameron Cooper, D.C., C.C.S.P.
Copyediting by Shirley Coe
Proofreading by Rita Sanel and Jasmine Star
Cover design by Toni Tajima
Book design and composition by BookMatters, Berkeley

First edition published by the Nourishing Company, 2000 (ISBN 0-9672718-0-0).

MediHerb product descriptions reprinted with permission from MediHerb Pty Ltd.

Library of Congress Cataloging-in-Publication Data

Levin, Pamela.
  Perfect bones: a six-point plan for healthy bones /
Pamela Levin.
    p. ; cm.
Includes bibliographical references and index.
  ISBN 1-58761-159-7 (alk. paper)
  1. Osteoporosis—Prevention—Popular works.
2. Osteoporosis—Diet therapy—Popular works.
[DNLM: 1. Osteoporosis—prevention & control—Popular Works. WE 250 L665p 2002]
I. Title.
  RC931.O73 L48   2002
  616.7'105—dc21   2002007660

Printed in the United States
First printing, 2002

1 2 3 4 5 6 7 8 9 10 — 06 05 04 03 02

In gratitude to the One who nourishes all.

CONTENTS

FOREWORD

EVERY ONCE IN A LONG WHILE, one comes across a health book that shows an acute understanding of the workings of illness. The illness's external manifestations are rightly interpreted and treated as signs and symptoms of an underlying metabolic disorder, one that is enmeshed in a complex web of interconnected bodily functions. Treating signs and symptoms is not the same as treating disease, but finding and correcting this underlying metabolic imbalance provides the surest road to success in many health matters. As Pamela Levin demonstrates in *Perfect Bones*, though the road may be difficult and long, the results are well worth the effort.

Identifying and untangling the various factors of bone health is a challenge that requires rare intellectual rigor and intuitive insight. It is more than just a skill; it is an art. In *Perfect Bones*, Pamela Levin meets this challenge. She understands and beautifully explains bone structure and metabolism, connective tissue biochemistry, and hormone balance, as well as the necessity of trace minerals, vitamins, essential fatty acids, herbs, sunlight, exercise, and balanced nutrition in maintaining bone health. The healing power of nature is awesome, but we need such guidance and commitment to make it a reality.

John R. Lee, M.D., 2002

PREFACE

EVERYBODY WANTS PERFECT BONES, yet fewer and fewer of us have them, especially as we age. Estimates say that in the next few years, forty-five million of us will be at risk for developing osteoporosis—a number expected to triple over the next sixty years, up to 135 million—and that more of us will die from osteoporosis-related problems than from the top two killers (heart disease and breast cancer) put together.

But it's not only adults—even the next generation is affected. Experts are currently lobbying the World Health Organization to have osteoporosis declared a pediatric-onset disease. Can anything be done? Is good bone health simply luck, or fate, or some big secret known only to a select few? Must we simply resign ourselves to this awful, debilitating, and ultimately fatal condition?

The premise of this book is that we can, indeed, do a great deal, that the power to have healthy bones is in our own hands, and that the choices we make on a daily basis are central to the outcome for our bones.

Osteoporosis has long been considered a disease, the inference being that it results from a body that simply malfunctions, as if such a breakdown were inexplicable and unstoppable. But if we view osteoporosis as a solution to a bodily problem, a demonstration of the body's natural healing ability, that hopelessness can change. Sick bones are the body's method of maintaining homeostatic balance in response to increasingly difficult challenges. Our bodies rob our bones of their life-giving minerals to supply these essential substances to areas that are more important for sustaining life, such as our heart and circulatory system. Thus, the key to maintaining healthy bones is to provide the body what it needs for homeostatic balance so it doesn't have to rob bones to sustain life.

How can we know if our bodies are out of balance and are, therefore, robbing our bones? Finding this out may seem a difficult task, for declining bone health has long been labeled a "silent disease." Yet after completing minimal research, I uncovered eighty-four separate clues that indicate when the body is robbing our bones to keep us alive. (See chapter 1.)

Perhaps we need to rename this silent disease the "deaf ear" disease, and conclude that we need to learn, or rather, relearn how to listen for it.

The National Osteoporosis Foundation has declared that the number one task in stemming a tidal wave of sick-boned people is to prevent osteoporosis in the first place, and that the best way to do this is through diet. Indeed, our nutritional states are the very bones of bone health.

It has been my great pleasure to take up the mantle of nutritional journalist and gather within these pages the essence of how to achieve and maintain a health-conferring state of nutritional balance. The goal is to provide your body with a better way to maintain homeostatic balance than developing porous bones.

We have every reason to believe that the power is in our own hands to create osteoperfecta: perfect bones.

Pamela Levin, Ukiah, California, 2002

ACKNOWLEDGMENTS

MY DEEP GRATITUDE to those dedicated giants of clinical nutrition whose knowledge is gathered in these pages. From an earlier era, both Royal Lee, D.D.S., and Price Pottenger, D.D.S., stand out. From today, special thanks to both the genius and generosity of:

- Dick Versendaal, D.C., who created a systematized, simple, and highly effective way to tap into the power of nature to heal;
- Michael Dobbins, D.C., whose knowledge of nutritional functions and pathways is unparalleled;
- Kim Sperry, C.N.C., who developed the vegetarian protocols listed in these pages, who patiently shared her considerable knowledge, and who personally taught me clinical nutrition;
- Mary Jane Mack, R.N., who took me under her protective wing professionally and mentored me, and whose friendly knowledge, support, and expertise were a constant source of inspiration;
- Dan Newell, C.N., for his presence, availability, specialized knowledge, and willingness to consult;
- Bruce West, D.C., for sharing his extensive knowledge and experience with so many, and with me in particular;
- Lee Vagt, D.C., for his clinical expertise and for helping me begin my own healing path;

- Fred Ulan, D.C., for his knowledge of how to discover and remove bone robbers, especially toxic heavy metals.

I also owe a special debt of gratitude to: Hogie Wycoff and Nancy Ellis, for nurturing the writer in me; Richard Lind, for his wise counsel and unending faith; Linda Simone, who so generously gave of her skills and herself; Lynda Myers, for extending a friendly editorial pen to the initial draft; Stacey Johnson, for her faith and dedication; Rick Moon, for his reassurance and problem-solving proficiencies; Jack Howell, for his guidance and enthusiasm; and Laura Samartino, for her loving guidance and profound wisdom, which have been and continue to remain crucial to my well-being.

Thanks, too, to those who gave other forms of assistance when needed, each in a distinctive and decisive way: Jon Buis, Penny Neal, Barbara Minogue, Renée Rutledge, Carol Gieg, Oni LaGioia, Jennie Burnstad, Marie McGarity, Karen Warren, Gail Shahbaghlian, Joan, John, Enid Griswold, Renée Freeman, and Sally Kroon.

Last, a special debt of gratitude to Corey Cameron Cooper, D.C., C.C.S.P., for expert and timely technical and text editing.

PART ONE

Your Bone Health and Your Options

ONE

What Is Osteoporosis and Can It Be Reversed?

THE PAIN SEARED THROUGH MY BACK like a bullet ripping through my spine, and it knocked me to the ground as fast as a bullet would. One moment I was reaching for my handbag to board the last leg of a flight home; the next, I was on the floor of the airport lounge, consumed by painful back spasms so severe I was not only unable to get up, I was going into shock. But I had not been shot. Rather, my back muscles had suddenly seized up, pulling my spinal bones out of alignment when I reached for my bag.

How could this have happened to me? Resting safely in bed at home two days later, having been helped by friends living near the airport and their chiropractor, I had plenty of time to review my situation. I had noticed a certain tension during sleep. I'd dismissed this as relating to work conflicts. Then there were backaches, which I began noticing at age twenty-six. I'd assumed they were from lifting kids and gardening. Still, morning stiffness had progressed over the years so that it took considerable time to get out of bed. I had become used to ignoring it and would remind myself that I wasn't as young as I used to be and try to forget it. I decided I needed to get in shape. Preparing for a run one day, I leaned over to tie my shoes and my back seized up. I was unable to get out of bed for a week.

Other warning signs had been more insistent. Once, for example, I shattered a tooth while eating bean dip. I asked my dentist whether this might relate to calcium deficiency and received a negative answer. When a second tooth shattered, I received the same reply. One night after a fourteen-hour plane trip, I stretched in bed and ruptured a disc in my lower back. During my recovery, I made all kinds of promises to myself that if I ever got better I'd be a really good girl and exercise no matter what. Meanwhile I felt hopeless, like I was doing something wrong but didn't know what.

Well-meaning family and friends began assorted campaigns. "You have to exercise every day!" insisted one. But by now even walking could make my back seize up. A friend concluded emphatically, "It's all in your mind." I only felt more hopeless. I balked when a concerned relative insisted I get a consultation with an orthopedic surgeon. I'd seen what had happened to my own mother: five major back surgeries beginning in her mid-forties and over thirty years of unrelenting pain that the surgeries did not relieve. Failing to heal from the last surgical invasion, she continued to deteriorate until she finally died.

To placate my family, I agreed to an X-ray. After spending two weeks recovering from a bulging disc, I presented myself at the X-ray department. The technician instructed me to lie in the very position that I already knew was foolhardy for my back. I objected; he insisted. I protested; he grew testy. Finally, I complied, reinjured the disc, and spent another two weeks recovering. The X-ray results were inconclusive. Considering that I was nearing fifty, I thought this sounded positive.

But I didn't feel very positive about my impaired lifestyle. For example, I'd learned to avoid physical exertion before noon, especially leaning over to make the bed. As the afternoon progressed, my body seemed to relax somewhat, and I could increase my activity level if I remained cautious. But that meant drastically limiting the things I loved to do, trying to cram them all into the tiny window of opportunity near nightfall. And I felt so frail, like a leaf in the wind that could easily be blown away. I had even become fearful of walking in a crowd, afraid that someone would jostle me and I'd be injured. I was beginning to think that I should give up trying to have the life I wanted and just learn to "go gentle into that good night." Had I been a different personality or a different age, perhaps my experience would have been different.

It certainly was for Carol Gieg, a woman whose problems began in childhood. Activity had been such a large part of her youthful life that she either didn't listen to or denied any signals her body gave her that she was going over the edge of toleration. But what she did do was keep going. After all, she was a young girl and activity was her life. Kids have accidents sometimes; they fall, they bump, they get hit. But five fractures in six years? That became impossible to ignore. Her parents took her to doctors, but the problems persisted. As an adult, she sought medical help and continued her beloved activity. Then she broke her hip. Her age: twenty-two.

These two scenarios, Carol's and mine, are two versions of a story with the same title: osteoporosis. This is what it's like to lose your bones. Whether you decrease your activity to avoid injury or keep active and hurt yourself, the result is ultimately the same. Slowly and silently your options as a viable human are increasingly limited. Molecule by invisible molecule, atom by atom, you lose your membership in the vertebrate world. You are reduced to the realm of those undulant creatures adrift in the tides, for whom mere osmotic changes are a threat to existence, who are all nerves, jellylike. You no longer have any stamina because you have already exhausted all your energy for the day. You are incapable of self-defense other than

that of the mythical Medusa: producing such a fearful stare that anyone who looks into your eyes will immediately be turned to stone.

THE BONES OF THE PROBLEM

Are such accounts unusual or rare? The numbers speak for themselves. In the United States alone, out of forty-six million people over
the age of forty-five, it is estimated that twenty-five million are dealing with their own versions of this story. Some sources claim 80 percent of these are women, though an Associated Press story reports a
ratio of six female cases for every one male sufferer. The Osteoporosis
and Related Bone Diseases National Resource Center reports that "2
million American men have osteoporosis and another 3 million men
are at risk for developing the disease." They add that osteoporosis
"affects nearly half of all people—women and men—over the age of
75."[1] Indeed, in the United States, over 1.3 million fractures are attributed to osteoporosis each year.

According to the Osteoporosis and Related Bone Diseases National
Resource Center, this debilitating disease afflicts more women than
heart disease, stroke, diabetes, breast cancer, or arthritis. Fully half of all
women between the ages of forty-five and seventy-five show signs of
some degree of osteoporosis.[2] Another report says that 35 percent of
women over age sixty and 10 percent of all men have osteoporosis.[3] A
pharmaceutical ad states that one out of every four women over fifty is
affected by osteoporosis.[4] In fact, a woman's risk of hip fracture is equal
to her *combined* risk of breast, uterine, and ovarian cancer. Statisticians
conclude that the incidence of osteoporosis is expected to increase
threefold over the next sixty years due to increased life expectancy, and
will cost the United States more than $10 billion annually.

Are these numbers inflated or unreasonable? Might they simply be
a miscalculation of demographic statistics? Unfortunately, no. Bruce

West, D.C., who has a long-standing clinical nutrition practice, concurs. "Most [adult] patients have osteoporosis," he says.

In the United States, the people who currently show signs of osteoporosis are only part of the picture, like the tip of an iceberg. Half the bone mass a woman loses over her lifetime occurs in the three to six years after menopause begins. Therefore, we can assume that the number of sufferers is growing dramatically since twenty million baby boomers have entered their menopausal years.[5] Some sources suggest that as of 2002, more than fifty-nine million women have or are at risk for osteoporosis. In the years after menopause, by age sixty-five or seventy, women and men lose bone mass at the same rate, and they can develop osteoporosis at the same rate. In 1995, author Gail Sheehy estimated that, before the end of the century, the number of people in the target age group (forty-five to fifty-four) would increase by one half.[6] However, even that turns out to be a conservative estimate. Current demographic research indicates that between 1990 and 2010, the number of women aged forty-five to fifty-four, the key menopausal group, is expected to grow by 73 percent. That translates to 3,500 women per day entering menopause and increasing their risk for osteoporosis.

Another part of this statistical picture, in a case of reverse sexism, is that men's bone health is often overlooked, partly because osteoporosis has been considered to be a disease largely affecting women. A second factor is that men frequently ignore and fail to communicate to their doctors the aches and pains often associated with the beginning stages of osteoporosis, and when they do, they may be ignored. Third, the incidence of prostate dysfunction and disease is rapidly increasing, with testosterone production often affected as well. Fourth, medical treatments often negatively affect testosterone levels. And for men, healthy testosterone levels are essential for healthy bones.

In the United Kingdom, The Royal College of Physicians reports that "the incidence of hip fractures rose 254 percent between 1954 and 1983 and was then still rising. . . . Every ten minutes someone in the U.K. has a fracture."[7]

In 1996, osteoporosis caused over twenty thousand hip fractures and twenty-four thousand forearm fractures in Australia alone. Now that number has increased to seventy-three thousand osteoporosis-related fractures per year, with the risk of dying from a hip fracture equal to that of dying from breast cancer. That's about twice the risk of getting cervical cancer. It is expected that more than half of all Australian women over sixty and one-third of all Australian men will be affected by this debilitating and death-producing problem.[8]

Worldwide, osteoporosis is estimated to affect two hundred million women. If men are affected at the ratio of one man for every six women, then thirty-three million men are also losing their bones. Over age fifty, men's risk of suffering an osteoporosis-related fracture is greater than that of developing clinical prostate cancer, and one-third of those men who have a hip fracture will die within a year. Studies of osteoporosis in men have found that "In 1990, 30 percent of the 1.7 million hip fractures worldwide occurred in men. By 2025, the total number of hip fractures in men will be similar to the current number reported by women. The complications and death caused by hip fractures is three times higher in men than women. The incidence of fractures in men is similar to that of women who are five to seven years younger."[9] Clearly, this is not only a "women's disease."

Even the next generations are being affected. The University of Colorado, for example, is seeing so many signs of the disease in children that they are recommending that the World Health Organization declare osteoporosis a pediatric-onset disease.

What is going on?

Two hundred million bodies worldwide are undergoing a long, slow process known as demineralization, or loss of the mineral content that gives bones their strength, which leads to porous bones. For many people it began long before midlife. However, in midlife the results are sufficiently manifest to see the effects of the erosion.

While the word "demineralization" might sound innocuous enough, a diagnosis of osteoporosis can arouse bone-chilling dread. Simply put, osteoporosis means losing your bones. So what does this mean to you, you might wonder? In a word, everything.

Bones comprise 10 percent of your body. Essentially unseen, bones form the very essence of your human shape. Perhaps if bones were on the outside of your body, like the exoskeletons of lobsters or crayfish, you would stay cognizant of their relative state of health or disrepair.

But bones don't just provide a structure for flesh and organs, they are dynamic and alive. Their living tissue is composed of minerals, the levels of which fluctuate under the influence of other body functions.[10] Like tree branches that provide a home for leaves and fruit and carry essential nourishment to them, your bones provide a home for your flesh and organs and store nourishment for them.

A bone's living tissue is composed of three parts. The outside is hard, dense bone, analogous to tree bark, where calcium is stored in large amounts. The second layer is soft, spongy bone. The third layer is like the sap of the tree: it contains marrow, which manufactures the red blood cells that carry life-giving oxygen to every other cell in the body. Without that oxygen, all the rest of the body's metabolic fires could not burn, and would smolder and suffocate. Even a slight tamping of the bone marrow's manufacturing process can cause the lassitude and exhaustion we intuitively call "bone tired."

Bones have a detoxifying function in the body, too. Harmful elements such as lead, radium, fluorine, and arsenic are removed from circulation and stored in bones and teeth.[11]

The red blood cells in the bone marrow are an integral part of the immune system. The marrow also manufactures antibodies, the white blood cells so small that a thimble can hold a quintillion. They patrol the borders of the body to keep out or neutralize invaders. Bones serve an additional health function crucial to the entire body: they store vital minerals needed to produce the enzymes on which every cell in the body depends.[12]

Strong bones are required for muscles to do their work. The ability to do anything—to act, to have strength—requires, first and foremost, healthy bones.

Because bones also record the body's history, they are the focus of fields of study and research such as bioarcheology, forensic anthropology, human osteology, and environmental archeology. Bones are the last human remains to decay, and whether they are well or poorly preserved, they chronicle stresses, physical hardships, and environmental pressures. According to the Museum of London Archaeology Service, long after you have left your bones behind, some future osteologist several thousand years from now will be able to "read" them and tell your age, race, gender, stature, and individual pathology, and could even reconstruct a demographic profile of your now-ancient population. They will be able to tell your family identity, ethnic or social group, and interpret the nature of medicine you used and your level of hygiene. What we now know about ancient history—the era of the pyramids or even the Stone Age—was gleaned from bones. Osteologists looking at the bones of former slaves, for example, have told us these people worked so hard that their muscles pulled off their attachments to bones, along with pieces of bone, eventually killing some of them. So completely do bones reflect human existence that stories of ancient life can be reconstructed through excavated bones.

Bones tell the truth, even when it's different from what we want to believe. One truth they are telling us is that the bones of people of all ages buried three hundred years ago in England were in far better condition than those from skeletons today. Bones have also revealed that osteoporosis was relatively uncommon until after World War I. The bones of people in developing countries reveal that they have far healthier bones than our own, despite the fact that these individuals consume less calcium per day than the average American.

Obviously, then, having sick bones is not an inevitable part of the human condition.[13] Some experts report that the increase in osteoporosis is due to the fact that people live longer. That's a disempowering idea that leaves only two unacceptable options: die early or degenerate slowly. Luckily, there's a lot of evidence that suggests the increase in osteoporosis is due to lifestyle, such as poor diet, bad food supply, an increase in hysterectomies and orchiectomies, and birth control pills. There are many empowering actions that can promote the possibility of living long and of staying healthy. The first of these is to listen to bodily signals.

HOW TO LISTEN FOR THE SILENT THIEF

So what are your bones telling you right now? Are they sending a message that creeping exhaustion and a vague ache reflect a silent thief at work deep inside you, stealing away your very bones? How do you detect the presence of such an invisible process now, while you can still do something about it? For most people, a kind of physical mousiness is a first indicator that the fate of the jellyfish might loom in their future. If that seems like little to go on, you're right. Osteoporosis is not called the "silent disease" because its onset is obvious. You'll need to review the at-risk factors listed below, which are compiled from a variety of sources, to get a better idea of your bone health.[14]

Warning Signs

- Feel depressed[15]
- Regularly consume white flour and/or sugar
- Consume soft drinks
- Have soft teeth
- Habitually overeat
- Have a tight jaw, clenched teeth, and/or teeth grinding
- Have receding gums
- Have periodontal disease
- Have loosening teeth in jawbone sockets
- Have eroding jawbone
- Have shifting dental plates (indicating further jawbone erosion)
- Have shattering teeth
- Have tooth plaque
- Wake up stiff in the morning
- Feel as if your body lacks solidity or substance
- Have weak muscles
- Lack fitness
- Feel physically fragile and fear getting bumped or jostled
- Suffer from pain in bones, especially in lower back
- Have joint tenderness or inflammation
- Have a tendency to cramp in legs, feet, or toes, especially at night
- Experience extreme fatigue
- Have heart palpitations
- Experience hot flashes
- Have brittle or soft fingernails
- Have premature gray hair
- Eat a diet high in salt
- Have unusually lean, low body fat
- Exercise immoderately (with second-degree amenorrhea, called athletic amenorrhea)

- Are over fifty
- Are nulliparous (no children, for women)
- Have a history of anorexia nervosa, overdieting, bulimia, or being thin
- Experience early (before age forty-five) menopause
- Have a stooped posture, forward bending of the spine (dowager's hump)
- Have transparent skin
- Are declining in height (an average of 1.5 inches every ten years after menopause; a loss of one-half to one inch in a year is considered diagnostic)
- Have low peak bone mass in early adulthood, or small, fine bones
- Suffer from prolonged immobility due to paralysis or illness
- Suffer from fractures, especially on the wrists, forearms, and hips, including vertebral crush
- Eat a high-protein diet, especially based on meat rather than vegetables and whole grains
- Drink fluoridated water
- Have a genetic predisposition, especially if fair skinned, small boned, with a family history (especially of osteogenesis imperfecta, a rare condition), of northern European or Asian extraction, female gender

Disease History

- Chronic renal (kidney) disease, including kidney stones
- Chronic liver disease
- Hypogonadism (male or female sex organs don't produce high enough sex hormone levels)
- Hyperthyroidism (thyrotoxicosis)
- Adrenal overactivity (Cushing's syndrome)
- Parathyroid overactivity (called hyperparathyroidism)

- Other endocrine diseases
- Rheumatoid arthritis
- Chronic lung disease
- Some forms of cancer, especially myeloma
- Rickets

Surgical Procedure History

- Removal of the ovaries
- Removal of part or all of the stomach or intestine
- Removal of the uterus
- Removal of the prostate
- Gall bladder dysfunction or removal

Drug History

- Anticonvulsants
- Corticosteroids (used for asthma or rheumatoid arthritis)
- Anticholinergics
- Certain diuretics (loop diuretics, e.g., furosemide; Lasix and thiazides)
- Anticoagulants (such as heparin or coumadin)
- Antibiotics, especially tetracycline
- Too high a dose of thyroid hormone replacement
- Antacids containing aluminum
- Phenothiazine derivatives
- Lithium
- Certain cancer chemotherapy medications
- Radiation exposure, including from medical treatment

Other Factors

- Estrogen deficient (postmenopausal or surgical menopause)
- Testosterone deficient (for men)

- Inadequate dietary calcium
- Insufficient exposure to sunshine resulting in inadequate levels of vitamin D
- Smoke cigarettes
- Lack exercise, sedentary
- Ingest caffeine, especially if excessive
- Ingest alcohol

Related Conditions

- Allergies
- Frequent colds and infections
- Gallstones or kidney stones
- Cold sores or herpes
- Mitral valve insufficiency or prolapse
- Arthritic or bony spurs

Any one of the above factors is sufficient to signal risk of osteoporosis; the more factors, the greater the risk.

Now that you've checked these warning signs against your own experience, you may feel concerned that you're losing your bones. Maybe that's true. But please, remember that the situation is not hopeless. You do not have to sit passively while you turn into a jellyfish.

How do I know? I know that there are effective choices because I recovered my bone health, and so have many others. You are assessing your situation now, and the sooner you become aware of it, the easier it will be to do something effective about it.

The collective experiences and research of patients and health practitioners indicate that bone health is linked to the health of the whole body, which is designed to maintain homeostasis, or a balanced state of health. From this perspective, osteoporosis can be seen as a biological *solution*: the body's attempt to maintain this life-giving balance in the face of some formidable challenges. For this reason, many health practitioners, including myself, have concluded that bones want to be healthy and will move into a more healthy state when provided with what they need to do so.

The rest of this book details what we have learned about bone health and how to recover it.

When Bad Bones Happen to Good People

Why are some people at greater risk of having their bones become porous and osteoporotic than others? After all, every human body is designed to have 206 bones, and every human body is designed the same way. Too, everyone's bones are composed of the same three parts described before: the tough, outer layer; a spongy, middle layer; and a center containing marrow. Isn't it odd that osteoporosis is not an equal opportunity disease? For example, if it's true, as studies suggest, that bone mass peaks between ages thirty and thirty-five and declines thereafter, and that women typically undergo a 30 to 40 percent bone loss between ages fifty and seventy, wouldn't it follow that every woman would be stooped over and unable to function by her seventh decade?

The answer to that last question is undeniably no. And one of the first factors that shows up to separate the lucky from the unlucky, of all things, is race. British author Clare Dover explains:

> When human life first emerged in the Rift Valley of Africa two
> hundred thousand years ago, we came with skeletons which
> were heavy and dense and extremely powerful. However, as our
> ancestors migrated, moving up the globe into higher latitudes,

genetic changes took place which caused deterioration in the
quality of the human skeleton. The European and other lighter
skinned races became lighter boned . . . black women of African
descent do not get osteoporosis with anything like the severity
of white women. They are the inheritors of the original human
skeleton . . . in adolescence black children are laying down an
additional 34 percent of bone, [while] white children are undergoing an average 11 percent increase.[1]

Nonetheless, 10 percent of African-American women over age fifty
have osteoporosis, and an additional 30 percent have low bone density
that puts them at risk of developing osteoporosis.[2] Naturopathic
physician Peter D'Adamo, N.D., has studied this phenomenon in
depth as he has worked to find the links between blood type and the
incidence of certain diseases. He, too, saw this pattern:

The movement of the early humans to less temperate climates
created lighter skins, less massive bone structures, and straighter
hair. Nature, over time, reacclimated them to the regions of the
earth they inhabited. People moved northward, so light skin
developed, which was better protected against frostbite than
dark skin. Lighter skin was also better able to metabolize vitamin
D in a land of shorter days and longer nights.[3]

Another factor crucial to whether or not a woman will develop
osteoporosis is how much bone mass she developed before the menopausal decade. Studies have shown that:

Total bone calcium in women increases from about 25 grams at
birth to about 390 grams by age 10, requiring an average retention of 100 milligrams of calcium per day during childhood (one
gram is about 1/30th of an ounce). With adolescence bone

calcium more than doubles, reaching 800–1000 grams by age
18–20. At the peak of adolescent growth, bones require daily
retention of 350–400 milligrams of calcium.[4]

Then, around age thirty to thirty-five, both men and women begin to
lose bone at the slow rate of "about .3–.5% per year."[5] In the five to
ten years after menopause, women lose about:

> 15% of their total skeletal mass. . . . Current medical research
> suggests that bone loss is going to occur after age 40, regardless
> of what we do. . . . If we can achieve the greatest amount of bone
> strength and density in the years between 25 to 40, then our
> bones can afford to lose some density with age without risking
> fracture or disintegration.[6]

As Dover points out, by the time fractures actually occur:

> The skeleton may have lost 30 percent of the calcium that should
> be its source of strength. . . . When several vertebrae have col-
> lapsed, there is a loss of height because of the shortening and
> compression of the spine. This reduces the capacity of the chest
> and abdominal cavities and interferes with the action of the
> heart, lungs, stomach and bladder and can cause difficulties
> in breathing, hiatus hernia and incontinence. The catalogue of
> suffering extends far beyond broken bones.[7]

These studies seem to be saying that to prevent problems in the
later phases of life, one must have had the forethought, first of all, to
have been born dark skinned, and secondly, to have made really
strong bones as a child and an adolescent. Since it's too late for all of
us to change the first and too late for most of us to change the latter,
what can be done? Is the situation really that hopeless? Not according

to my experience or the experiences of other people who have addressed the roots of their bone weaknesses, as we shall see.

YOUR BONE BANK

The analogy of a bone bank is useful to better understand what happens in osteoporosis. Each person has a bone bank account that was opened during fetal life. Deposits are made and maintained in this account at a brisk pace during childhood and adolescence when growth is rapid. Everyone can make deposits and withdrawals. In osteoporosis, for whatever reason or reasons, withdrawals occur at a far more rapid rate than deposits. If the account had plenty to draw on in the first place, the symptoms of osteoporosis won't show up for quite a while. But if the account had little surplus, any slight increase in withdrawals can jeopardize the account. In this respect, osteoporosis is a symptom of bone bankruptcy.

Bone bank deposits are made, kept, and withdrawn through a cycle of metabolism that continuously forms, maintains, and breaks down bones. If you are dark skinned, you have a genetic advantage in that you have substantial deposits in your bone bank to begin with, so you can afford more withdrawals before reaching a danger point. Also, adult men average more deposits than adult women. In part, this is because men lay down thicker bones during their bone-building phase and because women make massive bone bank withdrawals to sustain pregnancy and lactation. Nonetheless, no matter what your genetic background or gender, imbalances in the metabolic cycle can produce osteoporosis.

You already have a bone bank account, and your body has been making deposits, holding resources, and making withdrawals all your life. No matter what the current state of your account, the Six-Point Plan for Healthy Bones will teach you how to manage this bodily bank account just as you'd manage any other investment, such as real estate, a retirement fund, or a stock or bond. Managing your bone bank so you'll have sufficient resources for your retirement years is both an accurate parallel and a healthy goal. To accomplish this, you only need to consider six basic points.

THE SIX-POINT PLAN FOR HEALTHY BONES

The components of the Six-Point Plan for Healthy Bones are:

1. Healthy connective tissue
2. Sufficient minerals and their vitamin helpers
3. Essential fatty acids and the ability to metabolize them
4. A balanced hormonal system
5. Proper digestive, eliminative, and muscular activity
6. A clean environment and healthy immune system

Every one of the six points (which are explained in depth in part two) is essential to bone health. Each point plays a crucial role in the cycle of making bone bank deposits, helping maintain them, or permitting withdrawals so the body can support cell activities everywhere. In turn, each point is central to the health of the entire body.

The first two of the six points deal with deposits. Instead of carrying in dollars and cents as in a monetary bank account, cells called osteoblasts transport deposits of collagen (connective tissue) and minerals. The connective tissue forms small fibrous beams that hold their payload of mineral deposits in beautiful crystals called calcium apatite, which are engineered like tiny bridges. In a bank, these would be made of steel and called safe-deposit boxes. In bone, they are collagen structures—connective tissues made of various proteins. A key to perfecting your bones, then, is to make substantial deposits of all the various components of collagen (Point One) and the minerals (Point

Two) needed to form crystal bone bridges. This is possible; the skeleton repairs itself with fresh calcium atoms every three months. In fact, 98 percent of the body's atoms are exchanged for new ones every year. A key to healing, then, is to take those atoms from top-quality food so the body can repair and express optimum health.[8]

The role of getting these deposits to the bank falls to the food group known as oils, or essential fatty acids (Point Three). They function like an armored vehicle that safely delivers deposits to the bank. Without these carriers, materials that bones need are left by the metabolic wayside, where they can eventually turn into roadblocks for other bodily processes. To get them out of the way, the body may put them in other tissues, causing soft, pliable tissues such as eardrums or the inside of arteries to harden. Or, the body may gather the minerals together to eliminate them, which may form stones in the gall bladder or kidneys.

The rate of these activities, whether to increase, hold, or withdraw deposits, is governed by hormones (Point Four). Pituitary, thyroid and parathyroid, adrenal, and gonadal hormones provide this direction in concert. For example, the cells that make bone bank withdrawals, called osteoclasts, have the role of reabsorbing and removing bone that needs repair. Far from being bad guys, these cells help keep bones healthy. They recognize places in need of mending, and they tear away any unhealthy bone. That makes room for osteoblasts to enter new deposits and restore health. The parathyroid hormone stimulates them to carry out this function, and the thyroid hormone calcitonin inhibits osteoblasts from making withdrawals. In women, these bone bank withdrawals are carried out at a much more rapid rate after the hormonal changes of menopause, but by about the sixty-fifth year, the rate for men and women is the same.

These glandular hormone factories cooperate; they pick up the slack for each other when necessary. However, if one of the hormone factories stops its contribution, another one can only substitute for a while, and then it, too, becomes exhausted. If nothing is done to correct the imbalance, the whole house of cards can eventually come tumbling down into a state of total bone bankruptcy.

The process of absorption (Point Five) determines what materials are made available to run these metabolic activities. The whole operation has to be kept moving along, with fresh supplies brought in and old materials eliminated as quickly as possible. If the process should bog down anywhere, the entire flow can back up, eventually shutting down everything.

The focus of Point Six is protecting this life-giving cycle of depositing, storing, and withdrawing bone mass. Thieves, robbers, and embezzlers, in the form of toxins, allergic reactions, and infections, skulk about, waiting to carry out their nefarious activities. The body must maintain the integrity of the bone crystals and their supporting structures and hold the bones' mineral treasure in the face of such attacks. Bone banks are vulnerable to robbery of their precious contents.

Some bone robbers arrive in the form of viruses, parasites, or bacteria that emit toxins that render the bone deposit boxes incapable of holding their priceless treasure. Other thieves create emergencies in various parts of the body, causing the hormones' directors to release bone deposits, making their riches available to fight invasion elsewhere. These messengers might say, "Never mind that your bones need these minerals to maintain their strength. Your heart needs them much more right now to keep beating, and if your heart doesn't beat, there's no reason to worry about your bones. Healthy heart contractions are much more important than healthy bones!"

Luckily there is a simple, natural solution to avoid bone bankruptcy, and that is to increase bodily investments. And the quickest, most effective method for doing that is to use organic whole foods concentrated to clinical potency to support specific organs or systems. That's money in the bank.

THE COLLECTIVE COST

The personal cost of osteoporosis means fearing that if you sneeze, or pick up a bag of groceries, or get jostled in a crowd, you'll fracture a bone. Once diagnosed, you face a life of declining health, bone fractures, unrelenting pain, and early death. But this profound suffering is not the only cost. What is the cost to society when bad bones happen to good people?

The statistics are staggering: Osteoporosis is responsible for more than 1.5 million fractures each year, including 300,000 hip, 700,000 vertebral, 250,000 wrist, and 300,000 other site fractures.[9] Many of these fractures result in long-term debilitation and unrelenting pain. In fact, one of every two women over fifty will suffer an osteoporosis-related fracture during her lifetime.[10] In the United States, forty thousand osteoporosis victims die within six months of their fractures annually. Fifty percent of all people who experience osteoporosis-related hip fractures never regain the ability to walk independently. Fifty percent also end up in nursing homes following a hip fracture. Indeed, more women will die from complications of osteoporosis than from breast and cervical cancer and heart disease together. In fact, the World Health Organization lists osteoporosis as the second largest world health problem next to cardiovascular disease. And the University of Colorado is campaigning to have osteoporosis defined as a pediatric-onset disease.

A full one-third of all American women will develop osteoporosis severe enough to cause a fracture, while it is estimated that at age sixty, a man has a 25 percent chance of breaking a hip or vertebra during his life. And, says Eric S. Orwoll, M.D., more men than women die after a hip fracture.[11] Indeed, he says, "One in every 8 men over age 50 will have an osteoporosis-related fracture. Each year, 80,000 men suffer a hip fracture and one-third of them die within a year."[12] In 1985, the national cost of these osteoporosis fractures was estimated to be $7 billion a year.[13] According to the U.S. Department of Agriculture, that figure was expected to escalate to $10.6 billion by the year 2000. In 1997, the figures for the year 2002, according to the National Institutes of Health, were even more staggering. "The estimated national direct expenditures (hospitals and nursing homes) for osteoporotic and associated fractures is $13.8 billion ($38 million each day) and the cost is rising."[14]

In the United Kingdom, the Royal College of Physicians found that patients with hip fractures occupied 20 percent of orthopedic beds, and that 80 percent of these were women over sixty-five years old.[15] In fact, the Royal College estimates that one in twenty men and one in four women over seventy have osteoporosis and will sustain a fracture related to it. And hip fractures lead to fatal complications in 12 to 20 percent of cases. According to Clare Dover, "Each year doctors in the UK see more than 60,000 hip fractures, 50,000 wrist fractures, 40,000 spinal fractures and about 50,000 other fractures related to osteoporosis."[16] The United Kingdom spends only £61 million on hormone replacement therapy, but problems caused by osteoporosis cost the Health Service more than £1 billion pounds a year.[17]

In Canada, the cost of treating femoral fractures alone exceeds $400 million per year. By 2010, the estimated cost of osteoporosis to Canada's health care system will be $1 billion annually.

Measuring the cost of osteoporosis by examining femoral fracture statistics reveals only part of the cost. The leading cause of death for women in America is reported to be heart disease, which at first may seem unrelated to osteoporosis. But the calcium the heart needs to continue beating, when not available from the diet, is borrowed from bones.

Once the bones are bankrupt of their calcium treasures (osteoporotic), heart failure is not far behind. Yet these deaths are reported as heart failure, not as end-stage osteoporosis, thus hiding costs that might be ten times more than those calculated using hip fracture statistics.

In America, death from osteoporosis is reported to be the twelfth leading cause of mortality. Yet only those who die due to complications from bone fractures and falls are counted in that number. Still, osteoporosis is estimated to cost the nation $3.8 billion.[18] And it will get worse. Why?

In addition to the twenty-five million people currently suffering from osteoporosis in the United States, twenty million baby boomers are entering menopause. Nine baby boomers are turning fifty every second, and there are seventy-six million of them altogether.[19] Demographers point out that by the year 2030, sixty-nine million of us will be sixty-five or older, with nine million being eighty-five or older. Sixty years from now, the number of people at risk for osteoporosis is expected to triple, in other words, to reach 135 million.

Eighty percent of those affected by osteoporosis are women (according to the National Osteoporosis Foundation), the usual caregivers of children, the frail, and the elderly. Who will be their caregivers? There will be fewer and fewer able-bodied caregivers for a population whose average age is getting older and older. The Chronic Care Consortium estimates that there are already ninety-nine million people in the United States today with chronic health conditions, and that number is expected to grow to 150 million by the year 2030. Clearly, osteoporosis is heralding a health crisis of societal proportions. Society simply does not have the resources to cope with this enormous problem.

But the cost of bad bones is not limited to middle-aged people. Two potentially life-threatening conditions in pregnancy have been shown to be preosteoporotic; in other words, to exist prior to bone bankruptcy. They are pregnancy-induced hypertension (high blood pressure) and preeclampsia (a toxic state in pregnancy that can lead to convulsions, coma, and death). These maladies affect one in seven pregnant women and are the leading cause of cesarean sections, pre-term births, and low birth weight babies, costing society billions of dollars. But that's just the beginning. Add the total cost of care for pre-mature infants in the United States, which is $20 to 40 billion per year. Then add the cost of hospital care of a low birth weight baby, which can run $7,000 per day, or as much as half a million dollars per infant.[20]

These costs don't take into account dental problems. It is unknown at this time how many dental syndromes, such as cavities or teeth cracking, shattering, wearing down, or becoming loose in their sockets, are the result of the body borrowing their calcium. Nor do these figures include any estimate of the cost of various immunologic disturbances.

In summary, a conservative estimate by the National Institutes of Health of the social cost in the United States alone (excluding statistics for dental problems, pregnancy and low birth weight babies, and heart problems) is $10 billion annually, a cost that is expected to double over thirty years.[21]

Clearly something must be done. But is help available? Let's turn first to the place most people go when they have a health problem: their local physician.

THREE

Bones Are Bones:
The Western Medical Paradigm

ASK FOR A DESCRIPTION of the typical osteoporosis sufferer, and you'll likely get a list with terms like: middle-aged or old woman, having a dowager's hump, slow moving, tired looking, hunched over, walks with a cane or walker, weak, has poor muscle tone, a resigned attitude, and depressed or downcast. Yet here came Carol Gieg to our first meeting, bouncing down the steps on a hot August afternoon. Her short shorts and halter top revealed a lean figure with the perfect muscle development of a world-class athlete. At five feet, five inches tall and 105 pounds on the cusp of turning forty, she looked to be in enviable physical shape.

As we settled into chairs in my office and began to talk, I soon discovered how wrong this impression was. Her first bone fracture occurred at age nine, she revealed. This was followed by a green stick fracture and a broken foot at age twelve, a dislocated shoulder at age seventeen, and a broken hand at twenty-three, facts she attributed at the time to being so active. But she'd also had only one period, at age sixteen, and none after that. By twenty-one, she began seeking a way to normalize this situation. Her first physician at the University of California in San Francisco was just beginning research on the links between fat and estrogen levels and osteoporosis. He conducted a variety of tests, and then told her not to worry. The next year, during a marathon race, she heard her hip break.

Still recovering, she turned to a second physician who put her on crutches, thinking it would rest her bones. It was a big mistake, she said, for her condition worsened.

A third physician put her on some hormones, including FSH (follicle stimulating hormone). A fourth one, a nephrologist (kidney specialist) studying the metabolic process in the kidneys, started her on estrogen. He also took a punch biopsy of the bone in her hip and sent it off to a fifth physician, a University of Kentucky specialist. His diagnosis came back: osteogenesis imperfecta tarda, a congenital bone disease causing the bones to fracture easily, for which there is little that medical science can do. Feeling hopeless, she gave up trying to get better and just tried to live with it.

Eventually the pain and discomfort became too much. This time she turned to alternative practitioners and a combination of massage, chiropractic, and a macrobiotic diet to ease the pain. Still, she was very fragile physically. Attending the University of California at Berkeley, where she was working on dual master's degrees in social work and public health, she kept a motorized scooter at each end of her commute train, where she would ride to school and park next to the building where her classes were located. No one knew her condition. Then she heard about the use of calcitonin injections for Paget's disease (chronic inflammation of the bones with thickening and distortion, also known as osteitis deformans).

Turning now to a sixth physician, she began calcitonin injections, only to become so sick to her stomach after each injection that despite her desire to regain her bone health, she eventually threw the drug away.

She met her seventh doctor during her work at a Bay Area children's hospital. She had now endured pain for ten years. The doctor told her unequivocally, "You have to gain some weight!" Conducting some lab tests, he told her that her immune function lab results were lower than those of a person with AIDS. Recognizing the truth in what he was saying, she gave up macrobiotics, concluding that it hadn't helped beyond giving her hope.

Then she heard of a physician who specialized in bone diseases at the University of Worster in Massachusetts and called this eighth doctor on the phone. He kindly consented to review her records, by now a pile of documents several inches thick. He called her back early in the morning on the Fourth of July and said, "You don't have OI (osteogenesis imperfecta); that was not a correct analysis, and the bone sample they took was too small to make a correct conclusion. You have severe osteoporosis." And he never sent a bill.

Relieved, frustrated, and confused, she widened her search and turned up a ninth physician; this one was in California specializing in using natural progesterone (see chapter 9). She began to use ProGest Cream made from Mexican yams instead of Premarin and Provera (synthetic chemicals that mimic natural hormones, see "Medical Treatment Approaches" below). She took a course in meditation and one in restorative yoga. She learned to breathe into the pain and relax deep muscle tissues that were constantly tense, and she finally began to gain some pain relief.

She next visited a tenth physician, a woman who gave her phytoestrogens and some herbs. That was followed by an eleventh physician, an endocrinologist who wanted to try kick starting her body's own estrogen production. She stopped all hormones, even avoiding the natural estrogens in soy products. By the second month, she had lost breast mass, had dark circles under her eyes, and felt awful. Unwilling to continue like this, she resumed ProGest Cream in a 10 percent concentration. In the first four years on ProGest Cream, bone density studies showed a slight increase in her bone mass. Then during her fifth year of use, when she was stressed at her job, she lost all the bone she had gained. Her last bone density study at the Osteoporosis and Related Bone Diseases National Resource Center revealed the same results: at nearly forty, she had the bone age of a seventy-six-year-old woman.

With such a history, I could see why Carol was so weary of searching for help. As a social worker who has spent her adult life helping people, she definitely qualified as a good person to whom bad things had happened.

THE MEDICAL PARADIGM AND YOUR BONES

Carol's ordeal is repeated thousands of times every day as osteoporosis sufferers search for answers. Their experiences demonstrate some of the basic principles that underlie current medical thinking about osteoporosis, namely that:

- Everybody's bones are the same.
- Everybody's osteoporosis is the same.
- Everybody's osteoporosis can be treated the same way.
- Appropriate treatment addresses symptoms rather than causes.
- Treatment consists of administering drugs until body parts are surgically replaced.
- There is no cure.

These principles are fundamental to a tradition of thought about disease that medical historian Harris Coulter, in his three-volume work *Divided Legacy*, calls the "rational school." Apparent in medical practice for two thousand years, the rational school uses logical analysis rather than observation and experience as the source of knowledge and studies disease entities rather than physical growth. It classifies common symptoms into disease entities, and once a hypothesis of causation is established, the rational school bases its treatment approach on chemical (drugs) or mechanistic (surgery) approaches that are designed to remove the symptoms.[1]

Most treatment for osteoporosis, therefore, consists of administering one or more synthetic chemicals to affect the course of the disease. Since the body operates on the principle that for every action there is an equal and opposite reaction, these chemicals have both a therapeutic effect and side effects, meaning results other than the therapeutic ones. For example, if a drug stimulates the body, eventually it will produce a letdown. The person first feels like they're getting better, but then they crash somehow or other.

With regard to osteoporosis, Alan Gaby, M.D., president-elect of the American Holistic Medical Association, summarizes the current medical viewpoint: "Conventional medical opinion is that osteoporosis is a relentless process that cannot be reversed and that the best we can hope for is to slow down the rate of bone loss."[2] John Lee, M.D., adds, "Present osteoporosis management emphasizes prevention rather than cure since true reversal has proven unobtainable by conventional methods."[3]

These are the beliefs that underlie the medical options that will be offered to osteoporosis sufferers. Let's now look at these issues more closely.

MEDICAL DIAGNOSIS OF OSTEOPOROSIS

Bone loss used to be diagnosed with X-rays, which don't show bone loss until 25 to 40 or even 50 percent of the skeleton has been depleted.[4] The primary tests now used to diagnose osteoporosis are bone mineral density studies (BMD). These use a radioactive photon beam; bone with greater mineral content absorbs more photons. Single photon tests usually check the wrist or heel bones. Dual photon absorptiometry tests (DPA) can check the hip or spine. The newer DEXA test, the dual X-ray absorptiometry test, uses X rays.

A DEXA test does not truly measure bone mineral density, but rather measures the amount of calcium in the body, which is a surrogate marker for bone density. It is less accurate, particularly in elderly patients. Thus, as stated on the Menopause and Beyond website, "Bone mineral density deviations are diagnostic guidelines, not treatment thresholds."[5] The medical community considers the DPA and DEXA tests to be state of the art for measuring bone loss.

The tests require expensive equipment that is unavailable in many areas. Typically, two measurements are taken a year apart to measure the rate of bone loss; each test costs around $200, and may or may not be covered by insurance.

If you are going to use these tests to track your bone health or the effectiveness of a treatment for osteoporosis, John Lee, M.D., recommends testing the lumbar vertebrae (the bones in your lower spine) rather than the usual trabecular bone (the spongy interior portion of the bone that's most susceptible to osteoporosis). He tells us that since lumbar bones are "relatively large and uniform, the test results are generally more clinically accurate."

He also advises that when having serial tests, "different techniques give slightly different results and, therefore, comparisons of test results using different techniques are not as good as using the same technique throughout. Further, it is wise to use the same equipment in the same testing facility, if possible."[6]

However, bone mineral density test results do not correlate directly with bone health. "Ideally," states J. C. Prior of the Division of Endocrinology and Metabolism at the University of British Columbia, the results of such tests "should be shown to correlate with the ashed

flexible - supple bones

mineral content of the bone, to parallel the tensile strength of bone, and predict the fracture frequency. None of the reported measurements can yet meet all these criteria."[7]

Indeed, according to J. E. Compston, from the Department of Medicine at the University of Cambridge, large increases in bone mass as seen in bone mineral density studies may actually be associated with reduced bone strength and unchanged or increasing fracture rates. In fact, says Kerri Bodmer, recent studies "indicate that fracture prevention is not necessarily associated with increase in bone density."[8] Truly healthy bones are not only dense; they are also flexible, supple, and strong as a result of healthy microarchitecture. BMD tests don't measure these characteristics, which correlate more with fracture rates than bone density. Bones that appear to be dense can actually be unhealthy—brittle, rigid, and prone to breakage. In fact, some medical treatments currently prescribed to treat osteoporosis cause bones to become more dense, therefore appearing healthy in BMD measurements, but actually becoming more dense and brittle, and therefore more prone to fracture. To be truly healthy, bones must be both dense and supple.

Another disadvantage of relying on BMD tests to determine bone health is that they only measure the density of one bone. But bones can vary in density from one to another. Also, calcium deposits may be thicker in one area, causing the machine to produce a higher density reading than is true overall. Additionally, test results are compared to the peak bone density of typical premenopausal women, not necessarily women in the patient's age group, thus discounting normal differences associated with age groups.

Some doctors and other health practitioners use tests that measure the levels of certain by-products of bone breakdown in the urine. These tests have several advantages: they might uncover bone loss in its earlier stages, before it manifests as a problem; they carry no risk of exposure to X rays or photons; and they are far less expensive than DPA or DEXA tests.

One such test measures calcium excretion in the urine as a marker for bone loss. However, results can vary by up to 50 percent from one day to the next.[9] And higher calcium excretion does not mean the calcium is being taken from the bone. For example, the body could be dumping calcium in conjunction with a high protein intake where the body is attempting to balance phosphorus.

At this point, normal lab values for people of different ages are not known, leaving the interpretation of these results a matter of opinion. Also, a great deal depends on when during the course of bone breakdown the tests are taken: urinary calcium is increased in the initial phases of bone depletion, normal later, and low when the bone bank calcium deposits are drained.

Another test that is useful for assessing bone loss measures something a DEXA test cannot, the rate of bone resorption. It provides a dynamic measurement of bone turnover. Whereas a DEXA test gives a semiaccurate picture of how much bone has already been lost, a bone resorption assessment provides immediate information about how quickly bone is being lost by measuring the amount of particular collagen (connective tissue) molecules (pyridinium cross-links and deoxypyridinium) in the urine. The greater the cross-link excretion, the more rapidly bone is being lost. Many practitioners now advise people who have already lost bone as demonstrated by a DEXA test to have a bone resorption test to find out their current rate of bone loss. Some researchers have found that the bone resorption assessment actually indicates fracture risk more accurately than bone density measures. The urinary test also allows for testing as often as desired. This urinary test is also useful for assessing the effectiveness of intervention strategies.

Measurement of a particular amino acid (NTx peptide) will soon be possible at home, using a device called the NTx Point-of-Care. It is

Bone Resorption urinary Test

a credit-card-sized device, prescribed by a doctor and purchased at a pharmacy, that measures how much of this by-product of bone loss is present in the urine.[10] Proctor and Gamble has purchased the device and tested it in Europe, with plans to expand to the United States.

Still another method for assessment, available in some practitioners' offices, uses ultrasound through the heel bone (calcaneus). Called an osteometer, this test creates a high-resolution image of the scanned bone.[11]

When doctors want to know the condition of different areas of bone, they may order a bone scan, which requires being injected with a radioactive dye or a bone biopsy, in which a hollow needle is inserted into the bone.

A test that is likely to be used far more frequently is for metabolic dysglycemia. It "alerts to early signs of glycemic and hormonal dysregulation that can lead to the myriad complications associated with type-2 diabetes. It is important to bone health because blood sugar control plays an important role in bone health, influencing how bones are built and broken down. Researchers have found that women with type-2 diabetes had a 22% greater likelihood of suffering a non-spinal fracture, despite having higher bone mass density than women without diabetes."[12]

MEDICAL TREATMENT APPROACHES

Once osteoporosis is diagnosed, what are the medical treatment options? Current treatments consist of administering one or more synthetic chemicals that block the body's ability to make bone bank account withdrawals. As J. E. Compston, of the Department of Medicine at University of Cambridge, summarizes, "Nearly all treatments available are antiresorptive."

However, each drug produces two reactions: a therapeutic effect and side effects. The long-term effects of new drugs are not yet known. If bone resorption is affected in some way, healthy bone usually compensates with a change in the amount of new bone formed. Thus it is theoretically possible that by reducing bone resorption, certain drugs could actually lower the rate of new bone formation, ultimately increasing the problem they were designed to treat.

Below is a list of the prescription drugs currently available, how they act to treat osteoporosis sufferers, and how each one works relative to the bone bank metabolic cycle of depositing, maintaining, and withdrawing. All are purported to slow down the course of the disease, not cure it.

Estrogen Replacement Therapy (for Women)

The original medical approach to osteoporosis was estrogen replacement therapy (ERT) (see chapter 9). Currently doctors in the United States prescribe $840 million worth of estrogen supplements.[13] ERT for postmenopausal women is based on the observation that bone bank withdrawals are made at a much more rapid rate when levels of estrogen are low. Apparently, low estrogen levels stimulate bone bank withdrawals: osteoclast bone cells speed up the rate at which they are reabsorbing bone (withdrawing from the bone bank). The idea is that increasing estrogen levels will slow this rapid breakdown rate.

Studies of ERT's effect on bone were originally conducted on women who were already severely osteoporotic, and ERT's effect on bone was measured by a decreased incidence of fractures. The role of estrogen in actually preventing bone loss before it occurs has not been determined, although it is widely prescribed for that purpose. John Lee, M.D., points out that the positive results seen in the bones of women who were already severely osteoporotic "fades in 5 years or so and, thereafter, bone loss continues at the same pace as in those women not using estrogen."[14]

Nonetheless, one in five menopausal women uses estrogen replacement therapy today. A recent report in *Women's Health Letter* observes: "Contrary to what hormone supplement manufacturers would like you to believe, the widely advertised health benefits of lower heart disease and osteoporosis risk with HRT [hormone replacement therapy] are not standing up to long-term scrutiny."[15] To summarize, estrogen replacement therapy does not help bone loss that has already occurred; however, it does slow the rate of bone loss, from 5 percent on average to 1 percent for women taking it in the first five years postmenopause.

Premarin is commonly used in ERT. In fact, it accounts for about 90 percent of the prescriptions for estrogen replacement ($672 million per year). William Campbell Douglass, M.D., states, "Unfortunately Premarin does *not* contain the same estrogen your body produces. Premarin is made from *horse's* urine and contains over 49 different horse estrogens, none of which is naturally found in humans. As a result, Premarin's effects on osteoporosis have been disappointing. What's worse, Premarin has a whole host of negative side effects, including physical addiction . . . and an increased risk of breast cancer!"[16]

Other side effects of ERT may include nausea, bloating, stomach cramping, vomiting, headache, breast tenderness and enlargement, water retention and edema, mood changes, vaginal bleeding, high blood pressure, and increased risk of uterine cancer.[17] Estrogen therapy has also been found to promote gallstones, rare liver tumors, and blood clotting. It is contraindicated in the presence of obesity, varicose veins, hyperlipidemias, fibrocystic breast disease, a history of breast cancer, endometrial cancer or uterine cancer, clotting disorders, or thromboembolism, liver disease, hypertension, smoking, and heart disease.

In addition to the side effects, some women refuse to take Premarin because its production causes great suffering to mares. They are first impregnated and then hooked up to catheter-type devices to collect their urine, which is made concentrated by keeping the mares dehydrated. Author and researcher John Robbins adds that they are also "forced to stand constantly on hard, cold, concrete floors, unable to take more than a couple steps, and are unable to lie down comfortably, for 7 of the 11 months of their pregnancy. Each year, 90,000 foals are 'disposed of' as an unwanted 'by-product.'"[18]

Other researchers have noted that the same therapeutic effect produced by estrogen replacement therapy can be produced by supplementing with 3 milligrams of boron per day so the body can make its own estrogen. (See chapter 9.)

Selective Estrogen Receptor Modulators

More recent arrivals on the market are the class of estrogen substitutes called selective estrogen receptor modulators (SERMS). They are "designer estrogens" (with the chemical name of raloxifene) that are hoped to mimic the good effects of estrogen, such as a lower risk of heart disease and stronger bones, while inhibiting any harmful effects, such as promoting uterine and breast cancer. One such product is Evista, marketed by Eli Lilly, which paid for a study that claims there was a dramatic drop in the risk of breast cancer in women who took it. However, the study did not state what the absolute risk for breast cancer was in those particular women in the first place. Also, the drug had almost no effect on the kind of breast cancer most commonly developed by younger women and those with a genetic predisposition to it (estrogen-receptor-negative breast cancer). And raloxifene increases the risk of serious blood clots.[19]

John Lee, M.D., described Evista as raloxifene, a chemical cousin of tamoxifen, which is prescribed with the justification that it causes a 55 percent decrease in the fracture rate. He said that these studies did not measure the big fractures that debilitate, but rather compression fractures, which are tiny bone fractures that you never know you have anyway. He added that Evista causes a 300 percent increase in strokes and that it does not relieve hot flashes. He said that women taking Evista get more flu and colds, and that women taking Evista have no reduction in hip fractures. He also stressed that Evista causes the buildup of a sticky gunk on the inside of the uterus that scientists are unable to identify.[20]

Raloxifene, according to Merck Pharmaceuticals, "acts like estrogen in the skeleton, guarding against bone loss, but blocks the growth-stimulating effects of estrogen in the breast and uterus, where hormone stimulation can lead to increased tumor development. . . . Preliminary results show raloxifene increases bone mineral density by 2 to 3 percent compared to a placebo and lowers cholesterol levels. Drawbacks associated with the drug include an increased risk of phlebitis, which is inflammation of the veins, especially deep vein thrombosis (conditions which precede one kind of stroke) and hot flashes."[21]

Progestins (for Women and Some Men)

Recently some doctors have begun to prescribe synthetic Progestins. These are chemical imitations of the natural progesterone that the body produces. The hormone progesterone has been shown to be far more important than estrogen for bone health; low progesterone levels mean reduced bone bank deposits. Dr. Lee states that a "lack of progesterone . . . causes a decrease in osteoblast-mediated new bone formation." Dr. Lee pioneered using natural progesterone creams for a wide variety of health problems (including premenstrual syndrome, fibrocystic breasts, fibroid tumors, ovarian cysts, endometriosis, and endometrial carcinoma). He stresses that "progesterone deficiency and estrogen dominance" are the problem in most of these health conditions, including osteoporosis. (For a list of the symptoms of estrogen dominance, see appendix III).

Excessively low levels of progesterone in a woman's body, he adds, are brought about by many factors, among them "nutritional deficiencies, stress, environmental xenoestrogens, toxins, follicular depletion, and of course, the hormonal imbalance induced by contraception pills composed of synthetic hormones."[22] Does that mean it's best to go get a prescription for synthetic Progestins? No, Dr. Lee states, "Provera, a Progestin that differs from progesterone by a methyl group at carbon 6, has also been found to provide modest increases in bone density but lacks the full biological generality of natural progesterone and is not free of worrisome side effects. Additionally, its monthly costs are approximately 10 times that of transdermal progesterone."[23] He adds, "It is a mystery to me why synthetic Progestins are recommended when the natural progesterone is available, cheaper and safer."[24]

One answer might be that some sources are claiming that you don't get a "therapeutic dose" using natural progesterone cream. In fact, however, the dose required is far lower when using the whole, naturally occurring complex.

Estrogen and Progestins in Combination

In addition to the risks for estrogen and Progestin stated separately above, side effects from combining the drugs include: nausea, vomiting, pain, cramps, or swelling or tenderness in the abdomen; yellowing of the skin or the whites of the eyes; breast tenderness or enlargement; enlargement of benign tumors of the uterus; irregular bleeding or spotting; change in the amount of cervical secretion; vaginal yeast infections; retention of excess fluid, which may worsen asthma, epilepsy, migraines, heart disease, or kidney disease; a spotty darkening of the skin, particularly on the face; reddening of the skin; skin rashes; worsening of porphyria, headache, migraines, dizziness, or faintness; changes in vision (including intolerance to contact lenses);

mental depression; involuntary muscle spasms; hair loss or abnormal hairiness; increase or decrease in weight; changes in the sex drive; and possible changes in blood sugar.[25]

In July 2002, an eight-year national study of hormone replacement therapy was canceled three years early when conclusive proof was found that long-term use of Prempro—the most popular brand of estrogen and Progestin in combination—increases a woman's risk of heart attack by 29 percent, stroke by 41 percent, and invasive breast cancer by 26 percent.[26]

Some of this was already known in 1995. In a study reported in *The New England Journal of Medicine* involving 121,790 women who used synthetic estrogens and Progestins to offset symptoms of menopause, it was found that these women also increased their chance of developing breast cancer by up to 40 percent after taking these synthetic chemicals for more than five years.

Testosterone

Although it is primarily used to restore the function of the vaginal mucosa and to increase libido in women, testosterone therapy has been used for both women and men with osteoporosis. It has been shown to increase bone density in those whose levels were too low and in some men with normal testosterone levels. The normal ovary produces some testosterone, and after menopause the adrenal glands provide some. According to Alan Gaby, M.D., "In women with testosterone deficiency, addition of testosterone to an estrogen regimen may provide added protection against osteoporosis."[27] Tablets taken orally are composed of methyl-testosterone. Side effects include acne and hair growth, and because testosterone is converted in the liver, testosterone tablets are sometimes not tolerated in people with low liver function.

However, synthetic hormones, whether they are Progestins, estrogen mimics, or testosterone substitutes, are chemical lookalikes—pictures of the hormones the body naturally produces. Because they substitute for real hormones, administration of any synthetic hormone can slow down or stop the body's own production, thus lowering the blood levels of the real hormone.

To determine current hormone levels, doctors may order blood tests, which are not necessarily accurate because they don't measure tissue hormone levels. Instead, John Lee, M.D., recommends getting a salivary hormone test. This can measure levels of progesterone, estrogens, and testosterone. Even if the person is already taking synthetic hormone replacement, the test reveals the amounts the body is actually producing because it only measures the hormones the body produces naturally. In other words, salivary analysis measures only bioactive steroid levels. Synthetic hormones bound inertly to carrier proteins are not bioavailable and thus are not accurate in assessing hormone levels in relation to bone loss. Nonetheless, most doctors are trained to use blood tests, however inaccurate, and continue to order them. This is another situation where it pays to be an informed consumer and find out salivary hormone tests results. (See chapter 9 to learn how to support the body in producing its own hormones; see appendix IV for sources for salivary hormone testing.)

The combined estrogen replacement therapy and hormone replacement therapy market is more than $2 billion per year in the United States alone, with a projected growth rate of 15 percent.[28]

Biophosphonates

These drugs are sold under the brand names Fosamax or Editronate, or generically as alendronate. (Other varieties now in development include Risedronate, Ibandronate, Zoledronate, Tibolone, Idoxifene, Lovermeloxifene, and Proloxifine.) Their action could be likened to having a chemical stop payment placed on some bone bank deposits so they can't be removed. To inhibit bone bank withdrawal, they bind "tightly to hydroxyapatite crystals [the collagen and mineral crystal deposits that make up bone] and inhibit bone resorption," according to Alan Gaby, M.D.[29]

Like the studies that demonstrated the positive effects of hormone replacement therapy, the tests for biophosphonates were conducted on women with existing vertebral fractures. A University of California at San Francisco study showed that "among women with existing vertebral fractures alendronate is well tolerated and substantially reduces the incidence of vertebral and clinical fractures including the incidence of hip fractures by about half." However, some of the studies defined "fracture" to include the many hairline fractures that occur over time and create no symptoms or problems.

Officially, the long-term risks and side effects of biophosphonates are said to remain largely unknown because Fosamax has just been approved by the FDA and physicians are just beginning to prescribe it. Currently side effects stated in the product information include nausea, and esophageal and stomach irritation; abdominal pain; bone, muscle, and joint pain; headache; heartburn; an altered sense of taste; and sometimes allergic reactions. Biophosphonates should not be used if blood calcium is low or if the person is on hormone replacement therapy or has kidney problems. The first generation of biophosphonates had adverse effects on bone structure.[30]

A study reported in *The New England Journal of Medicine* in February 1998 reported that Fosamax takers showed an average bone density increase of 3.5 percent at the spine and 1.9 percent at the hip, a fact that sounds impressive until compared with magnesium studies that show an increase of 8 percent. In fact, in one study, fifteen of nineteen women had spinal bone mineral density readings below the fracture threshold; after a total dietary program emphasizing magnesium instead of calcium, "within one year, only 7 of them still had BMD values below that threshold."[31] That's one reason the *Women's Health Letter* recommends trying magnesium supplementation first (see chapter 7). According to Kerri Bodmer, another reason is that "Fosamax is so disruptive to the gastrointestinal system that it must be taken at least 30 minutes before the first food, beverage, or medication of the day. . . . Then, you aren't supposed to lie down for at least 30 minutes and until after you've eaten. Fosamax actually works by interfering with the body's natural bone resorption process, and by doing so can lead to other serious health risks."[32] Biophosphonates such as Fosamax accumulate in the skeleton, where they remain for long periods of time. The long-term effects of such accumulation are unknown.

Editronate, like Fosamax, is a biophosphonate. It was approved because two studies showed it increased bone density and decreased new spinal fractures for people who used it for two years. However, a three-year study shows no difference in the rate of spinal fractures between those who took it and those who didn't. Even though it's been shown to produce denser bones, Editronate unfortunately also makes them softer (osteomalacia) rather than stronger.[33]

These facts were revealed in research on biophosphonates at the Department of Medicine at the University of South Carolina, which reports that these drugs inhibit osteoclastic (cells that resorb bone) bone resorption at lower concentrations. However, at higher concentrations they may "inhibit mineralization and cause osteomalacia," a disease in which "the bones soften so that they become flexible and brittle and cause deformities. It is attended with rheumatic pains. The limbs, spine, thorax, and pelvis especially are affected; anemia and signs of deficiency disease present; the patient becomes weak, and finally dies from exhaustion."[34] The research was reported by N. H. Bell and R. H. Johnson. They add that "bone formation is also reduced as a consequence of diminished bone resorption." In summary, because biophosphonates block bone resorption, they "come with the risk of actually impairing other important aspects of our health."[35]

John Lee, M.D., reports that biophosphonates such as Fosamax or Editronate are made from the ingredients used in bath tub cleansing powder to clean the skin cell scum off the tub (phosphonate). They are used for this purpose because they dissolve human cells, which is why, if the pill stops somewhere after being swallowed, it will burn a hole through the esophagus or stomach. Their effect is to poison the cells that resorb old bones. Therefore the bones become more likely to break the longer the drug stays in the body; the drug has a negative effect on the tensile strength of bone, ultimately causing it to break. Biophosphonates block all new bone formation, thus causing bones to become older. Studies of the first years of taking one of these drugs don't show these bone problems because bones are replaced very slowly. It's only after five or so years of taking biophosphonates that the fracture rates begin to increase. Initially the drugs are picked up by the bones, but the body doesn't know how to get rid of them; therefore, they have a half life in the body of fifteen years, meaning it takes the body fifteen years to eliminate half of the drug.[36]

Dr. Lee adds that no study has shown hip fractures to decrease as a result of taking this class of drug. Studies have only demonstrated a decrease in the tiny compression fractures that don't cause problems, the ones that have no clinical significance and are generally undetected. It is for these lesser fractures that the companies can claim their drug reduces the fracture rate. Dr. Lee declares that Fosamax has been shown to cause an increase in bone mass of 2 to 3 percent, which, when 50 percent of bone has been lost, is nothing. "Fosamax doesn't work," he concludes, adding that natural progesterone has been demonstrated to cause a "15 percent or more increase in bone mass in two years."[37]

Calcitonin

The brand names for calcitonin are Calcimar and Cibacalcin. These drugs are a synthetic chemical imitation of the calcitonin hormones produced by the thyroid gland. The body's natural hormone helps regulate blood levels of bone-building calcium and reduce the rate of bone bank withdrawals by inhibiting bone-destroying cells. According to Alan Gaby, M.D., "Calcitonin is a potent inhibitor of osteoclasts, the cells that cause bone resorption."[38] "When injected into humans," states John Lee, M.D., "there is a brief period of new bone formation. With further sets of injections, the bone response becomes progressively less. When discontinued, the benefits gained are quickly lost."[39]

Formerly, the synthetic chemical version was injected daily at a doctor's office; however, it is now available in a nasal spray (Miacalcin). It works as an antiresorptive agent and is for people whose bone density is already low but whose rate of bone turnover is high.

Nausea, rhinitis (inflammation of the nose with the nasal spray), and arthralgias (joint pain) are common side effects of synthetic calcitonin.[40] Other side effects, writes Alan Gaby, M.D., "include transient facial flushing, nausea with or without vomiting in about 10% of cases ... [and rarely] severe allergic reactions, including anaphylactic shock [an acute, life-threatening form of shock resulting from an allergic reaction], and one death due to anaphylaxis." Dr. Gaby concludes, "At a cost of $7.50 per day (or more than $2,700 per year), calcitonin is probably the most expensive treatment for osteoporosis."[41]

Sodium Fluoride

This chemical has been put on teeth to reduce cavities and added to drinking water. It is now in development in a slow-release form for treatment of osteoporosis because it is purported to build new bone bank deposits, thus preventing fractures, when used in conjunction with calcium citrate. Citrate is a salt of ester of citric acid, which is a white, crystalline, water-soluble powder used to flavor beverages, confections, and pharmaceuticals. It is reported to be the only widely tested drug that can stimulate new bone formation.

Apparently sodium fluoride makes bones denser so they seem healthier during bone density studies, but the resultant bone is less flexible, and therefore more likely to break. High doses of this drug were found to increase bone mass but also to impair bone strength.[42] John Lee, M.D., underscores that fluoride "may slightly increase the x-ray appearance of bone mass but the resultant bone is of inferior quality and actually increases the risk of hip fracture," whether that fluoride is from osteoporosis therapy or fluoridated water. "Fluoride," he states "is a potent enzyme inhibitor and, in bone, causes pathologic changes leading to increased risk of fracture. Fluoride, in all forms including tooth pastes, should be avoided."[43] Additional side effects may include nausea, vomiting, diarrhea, and leg pains. Alan Gaby, M.D., concurs: "Any potential benefit of fluoride treatment must be balanced against reports of serious side effects, including anemia, gastrointestinal symptoms, arthritis, and recurrent vomiting."[44] Indeed, states Michael Dobbins, D.C., "Fluoride is a highly toxic halogen."[45]

New Developments

Researchers continue to explore treatment possibilities for osteoporosis. New developments include:

Minocycline. This antibiotic has been shown to increase bone mass in laboratory animals and is now being tested on women. Researcher C. T. Liang showed that Minocycline, a tetracycline-like compound, "was as effective as estrogen in preventing a 15 percent bone loss in rats whose ovaries had been removed. Liang hypothesizes that the drug blocks the synthesis of an enzyme known as collagenase, which breaks down collagen. Collagen is a protein that paves the way for new layers of surface bone to form and serves as a protection against special bone-eating cells called osteoclasts. Without collagenases, the thinking goes, bone can form unmolested."[46] However, antibiotics also kill off the body's natural flora that help digest food and provide a protective barrier for the skin and gastrointestinal tract. Antibiotics interfere with absorption of the various vitamins and minerals necessary for healthy bones. The natural intestinal flora also manufacture vitamin K, an essential helper in maintaining bone health. Their absence sets the stage for osteoporosis because the rate of bone bank withdrawals is dramatically increased as the body leaches calcium from the bone.

Because the flora that help digest food have been killed off, food remains undigested and turns to poison in the body, and antibiotics weaken the immune system's defenses. Immune and other cells cannot get the nutrition they need to function properly when their work load is greatly increased due to having to clean up so much undigested food. Use of antibiotics has meant trading short-term help knocking out infections for long-term problems.

Antidepressants. Statistics have shown a correlation between depression and bone density, which is why drug companies urge physicians to encourage their patients to take antidepressants.[47] Depression can also be an indicator of hormone imbalances (see chapter 9). Depending on the kind, antidepressants have a variety of side effects, such as motor or cognitive impairment.

Cytokines. Researchers are also looking at cytokines, which bone marrow produces. They are encoded proteins that control immune activity within the cell or from a distance. Their tiny immunologic messages can mediate or turn on or off immune system defenses. Cytokines can contribute to bone loss when several kinds act in concert.

Anabolic Steroids. These are sometimes prescribed for men who have osteoporosis because they help build bone and muscle mass. One drawback for women is that they masculinize, meaning a women might develop a mustache and a deeper voice. They also increase the risk of heart disease and can be toxic to the liver.

Gamma-Pyrones. These drugs inhibit parathyroid hormone, but the number of people developing osteoporosis as a result of too much parathyroid hormone is probably quite small.

Ipriflavones. These are synthetic alterations of isoflavones, proteins found in soy. Some evidence suggests that higher intakes of iso-flavones are associated with denser bones.

Parathyroid Hormone Analogues. These are chemically altered substi-tutes for the body's own parathyroid hormone. One brand is Fortéo. It spurs the production of osteoblasts, the cells that stimulate bone growth. But the manufacturer (Eli Lilly) stopped a study on people after finding bone cancer in laboratory rats that were given high doses of the hormone over their lifetimes. Fortéo would seem to be most effective in people whose parathyroid hormone levels were low in the first place. (For protocols to support parathyroid hormone production nutritionally, see chapter 9.)

Vitamin D Analogues. Even though too much vitamin D can actually cause bone loss, recent ongoing research focuses on chemicals that are similar to vitamin D in function, but differ in structure. The goal is to create a patentable chemical that stimulates the cells that make bone bank deposits (in other words, an osteoblast-stimulating agent or enhancer).[48] (See chapter 7 for a discussion of the uses and dangers of vitamin D.)

Strontium Ranelate. Strontium is a bivalent metallic element whose compounds resemble those of calcium. In nature it is only found in the combined form. It is used in fireworks, flares, and tracer bullets while in its hydroxide form; it is also used in refining beet sugar.

Implanting New Bone. New bone cells are currently being grown on a glass-like material that "allows bone cells to grow and bond with each other quickly," according to BBC News Online. The glass acts as a scaffold onto which the bone cells cling and as a material to bind existing bone to the new cells. This will most likely find application in people with complex fractures. It is already used in dental surgery and bone surgery to fill holes and mend fractures. As with any technique where material is injected, infection is a risk.[49]

Genetic Research. Research is also underway to see whether gene modulation or splicing might slow, halt, or reverse bone loss.

According to IMS Health Inc., a research firm that tracks prescription drug data, the market for bone density regulators, not including hormone replacement therapy, totaled $2.4 billion in the twelve months ending June 2001.[50]

SURGICAL REPLACEMENT OF BONES

When bones wear down or break, surgical procedures can replace hip sockets, knees, or shoulder joints, and sometimes even provide new ankles, elbows, or finger joints. Currently about 125,000 Americans get new hips each year, and another 240,000 get their knees replaced.[51]

Called arthroplasty, the joint is surgically reformed using a ceramic or metal ball with a plastic cup, sometimes cemented into place. This option yields positive results for many people, which led Edith Crenshaw to request it.

Edith was seventy-five when her bone health came crashing down. "I had more and more difficulty with motion of my arm, particularly reaching it back to put on a coat. It got so bad I had trouble opening my purse, cooking, cutting bread, opening cans, and holding the newspaper, and doing needlepoint had long since gone by the wayside." Her internist said she had a frozen shoulder and recommended some exercises that she did faithfully. They didn't help.

A new physician took a lot of tests and said the same thing. Then an orthopedist said that she didn't have a frozen shoulder; she had erosion. "If you were younger and your livelihood depended on it," he said, "we'd do surgery, but it's a long climb up the mountain for a short ride, and we don't recommend it." After developing pain in her groin, she again saw an orthopedic surgeon. "He did the tests and said, 'We start the scale for hip surgery at 60 points and you're at 100, so you're a candidate for surgery.' I said, 'Hip surgery? What really bothers me is my shoulder!' So he checked that out. I was getting the pre-op lab work for the hip surgery when he came in and said, 'you need shoulder surgery.' I went home steaming."

Her daughter picks up the story. "It was supposed to be a two-hour surgery. After four hours I called, and they said not to worry, everything was fine, it would be another hour. After another hour and a half I called again, and they said the same thing and it would be another hour. Finally I said, 'This is not acceptable; I'll go to the operating room and get an answer myself, or else you go in and get a direct answer.' So five minutes later they called and apologized."

It turned out that as her mother's surgeon had carefully completed his final micro movements to reattach the last muscle to her now rebuilt shoulder, her entire shoulder bone shattered, leaving the count-less fragments in his gloved hand. Up until that moment, her osteo-porosis had gone undiagnosed.

Now seventy-six, Edith reports, "Once in a while I have really sharp pain in my hip, and limp, but it's very rare. I walk a lot better with a lot better mobility. I wouldn't go in for hip surgery now. I've been doing a lot of exercises, tai chi, and water aerobics. I'm sure I have osteoporosis. My shoulder was evidence of it. It's only a question of how bad it is. I still have residual pain. On X-ray my hip looks like my shoulder, but I don't have the mobility restriction that I had with my shoulder. The surgeon recommended extra calcium, so I take that, and chondroitin sulfate and glucosamine."

Although this combination will likely result in phosphorus and magnesium imbalances over time, Edith's doctor is beginning to address two points of the Six-Point Plan for Healthy Bones in recom-mending that she take extra calcium and products to strengthen her connective tissue. When I tested her during this interview (using the method described in chapter 4), I discovered that she was also low in certain essential fatty acids, Point Three of the plan. Without oils, the calcium would not make it to her bones no matter how much she takes.

Outcomes like these definitely reinforce the idea that it's better to get the body to repair its own bones whenever possible. But there's more. As orthopedic surgeon and author Jason Theodosakis points out, "Even with the new joint, you don't have as much function as you did before. . . . With surgery, there's always the risk of dying or becom-ing permanently disabled. And the surgery is painful, expensive, and not permanent—in ten years or so the replacement will begin to fail and the operation will probably have to be redone."[52]

Besides, significant bone bank capacity is also lost. The body can't use a titanium implant to store or borrow minerals like it can with a living bone. Bones repaired naturally are often even stronger than before, as evidenced by the increased strength of some bone fractures allowed to heal naturally.

TREATMENTS THAT DAMAGE BONES

Certain medical treatments for other conditions can set the stage for osteoporosis. In fact, some of the treatments now being offered for osteoporosis are damaging to bones. These include:

- Antibiotics.
- Anticholinergics.
- Anticonvulsants (used to treat epilepsy).
- Cisplatinum (used in treating cancer). It can cause excessive loss of magnesium.[53]
- Corticosteroids (used for conditions such as asthma or rheumatoid arthritis).
- Digoxin (used in heart conditions). It can stimulate magnesium loss.
- Diuretics. Some, such as Lasix and thiazides, increase blood calcium levels and can cause complications in conjunction with calcium and vitamin D supplementation. Others can increase calcium requirements.[54] Some (hydrochlorothiazide, chlorathalidone, furosemide) promote magnesium deficiency.[55]
- Glucocorticoid therapy (used in the management of symptoms of inflammation in collagen diseases, asthma, rheumatoid arthritis, and conditions of adrenal suppression, such as Cushing's syndrome). It is the most common cause of juvenile-onset osteoporosis.
- Indomethacin, ibuprofen, and other nonsteroidal anti-inflammatory drugs (NSAIDS) used for pain relief. These weaken the hip joints.

- Radiation exposure.
- Sodium fluoride. "Women participating in a study at the Mayo
  Clinic in Rochester, Minnesota, were three times as likely to
  suffer from a fracture of the arm, leg, or hip if they took sodium
  fluoride than if they took a placebo. Some of the participants
  also suffered from unusual lower leg pain, perhaps due to
  stress fractures," according to James Balch, M.D., and Phyllis
  Balch, C.N.C.[56]
- Thyroid hormone replacement. Too high a dose can stimulate
  bone loss.

Some surgical procedures can have bone-crushing effects. Common
surgeries that contribute to bone breakdown include removal of:

- Gallbladder (cholecystectomy)
- Ovaries (oophorectomy)
- Parathyroid
- Prostate (prostatectomy)
- Stomach (subtotal gastrectomy)
- Testes (orchiectomy)
- Thyroid
- Uterus (hysterectomy)

OTHER MEDICAL OPTIONS

Noticeably absent from these medical options is any mention of nutritional approaches, and one must wonder why. One factor is that doctors are not taught about nutrition in medical school. A doctor friend
of mine tells me that his entire nutritional education in medical school
consisted of one fifteen-minute segment of one lecture. Alan Gaby,
M.D., past president of the American Holistic Medical Association,
reports having been "told more than once in medical school to shut up

about that mineral and vitamin research stuff, never mind that it's published in medical journals."[57]

This mindset doesn't seem to be changing. Michael Janson, M.D., president-elect of the American College for Advancement in Medicine and president of the American Preventive Medical Association, reports that most medical schools still do not teach nutrition. Adds Jean Barilla, M.S., "Through the early 1980s no medical school in the United States required a nutrition class. Today, several medical schools have added nutrition courses, but most do not address disease prevention and management."[58]

Why is this? Funding for certain faculty positions, research projects, and education is increasingly under the control of pharmaceutical industry whose primary interest is seeing to it that new doctors use their products. They put their money behind research that's likely to lead to the development of patentable products. Nutritional products are not patentable because they are considered food, not medicine, so there is no profit in them. When companies find a food or herb that works, they produce a chemical alteration or make a chemical imitation of it, which is patentable, and then send their product representatives around to the doctors' offices with glossy literature and free samples to "educate" the doctor. For particularly profitable products, doctors are offered continuing education seminars in Hawaii, or Barbados, or Palm Springs, where they will further their "education" about the patented product for a few hours a day.

This state of affairs is enforced through binding doctors to a legal standard of practice. That means that if they offer something different than the other doctors in their area, they can be sued for malpractice and also have their license to practice taken away. So even if doctors are interested in nutrition and want to pursue it, they can be putting their careers and bank accounts on the line even by experimenting with it. This is true even though medical literature abounds with information attesting that nutritional approaches work. Most doctors follow the standard practice for treating osteoporosis, and the standard practice is limited to prescription pharmaceuticals and surgery. A suffering consumer who goes to a doctor expects to be presented with all the known options. But this is not the case; most physicians will only present the standard practice options.

Does the source of funding affect the outcome of a study? Seventy articles, reviews, and letters about calcium channel blockers were assessed for the author's position on the drugs relative to the author's financial gain from drug manufacturers. Authors who supported the drugs had from a 37 to a 96 percent financial connection with drug companies.[59]

"Interestingly, the people who researched these researchers do not believe that financial remunerations resulted in biased studies. We're not so sure about that," says the *Women's Health Letter*. "If you conduct a large, expensive study for a company that's either lining your pockets or financially supporting a great deal of research for your educational institution, would you say the drug is of little or no value? If you did, do you think you'd be asked to be part of a future research project from this manufacturer?"[60] Nonetheless, these same researchers often point a finger at nutritional information, saying it is inadequately researched, thousands of actual studies notwithstanding.

The government agencies that could do something effective to change this situation actually work to maintain the status quo. Various supposedly independent departments are actually under the indirect control of the pharmaceutical giants. These corporations give large donations to the election coffers of officials who are "encouraged" to vote in specific ways or to appoint certain people to key positions in the governmental agencies that make relevant policies. Such appointed officials often have worked for the pharmaceutical giants prior to their government jobs.

There is also, says Julian Whitaker, M.D., "an incestuous relationship between the F.D.A. [Food and Drug Administration] and drug companies. . . . Ambitious young ladder-climbers know that the best way to get high-paying jobs at the pharmaceutical firms is to put in their time working at the F.D.A."[61]

A treatment that becomes accepted as a standard of practice in the medical system is based on scientific investigation. This process, reports Dr. Dean Black, identifies large samples of patients who all suffer the same condition, standardizes treatments so no variation can exist from patient to patient, hypothesizes what will be found before finding it, holds confounding variables constant to keep them from contaminating the results, tests for statistical significance, replicates the research, and submits it for peer review.[62]

The pharmaceutical companies' control over medical doctors has been greatly aided by grants from the Rockefeller General Education Board and other foundations, which, since 1910, have sponsored so many grants to allopathic medicine that, in 1974, for example, nearly half of all medical school faculty received a portion of their income from foundation research grants, with over 16 percent being entirely funded this way. Researcher Barbara Griggs concludes that this has hardly been disinterested philanthropy, "since it eliminated all effective forms of alternative medicine for years, and promoted a monopoly medicine which is heavily drug-oriented."[63] This situation has been further reinforced by a decision by *JAMA*, the *Journal of the American Medical Association*, to accept advertisements for patent medicines, which supply more than half the A.M.A.'s revenue.[64]

So what is an afflicted person to do? Are there clinically effective options that are free of untoward effects and that help the body create perfect bones? States Alan Gaby, M.D., "While collecting articles over the years, I came across many that suggested there is more to osteoporosis treatment than calcium, estrogen, and exercise."[65] Indeed, the answer to this question requires a different paradigm with different ways of thinking about bodily processes and healing.

Carol Gieg experienced such a shift when she changed jobs. Leaving the hospital where she was formerly employed, she moved farther north in California and began work as a mind-body therapist. As part of her new job, she began visiting healers in the area on behalf of her patients. This led her first to a chiropractor who showed her how to stretch and break up scar tissue that had formed in her muscles. He also referred her to a nutritional counselor. Using the method described in chapter 4, the counselor recommended a clinical nutrition protocol (a plan including recommended supplements). Her counselor was one of my teachers, and she connected me with Carol to be interviewed for this book.

When I met with Carol, I found her well-informed and articulate, and also very skeptical of new treatments. After all she'd been through, I could see why she felt that way. Should she hope that, after two decades of searching, she might still find effective help? This was the dilemma facing her as she decided to be tested one more time to at least see what turned up. Using the same assessment described in chapter 4, we found evidence of weaknesses in all six areas of the Six-Point Plan for Healthy Bones.

This could be greeted as either bad news or good news: bad because so many things were out of balance and in need of correcting, but good in that there are proven nutrition protocols to address and strengthen each area. Clearly not one to give up easily, Carol decided to proceed, tackling the most important area first. We will follow her progress to see how she does.

It is hard to believe that a new way of thinking might yield an effective plan of action. I understood this well, for I, too, was skeptical when I searched for treatment for my condition. I was up to date on current medical options, and I thought that if I knew those, I knew

everything. Now, looking back, I am incredibly grateful that I followed clinical nutrition protocols in spite of the lack of support for
them from the medical paradigm.

You might argue that these new ways of thinking about healing are
unproven. Actually, there are thousands of studies published in
respected medical and scientific journals showing the benefits of clinical nutrition; yet these are largely ignored. Most of the treatments
physicians use every day are unproven, and some can even be haz-
ardous. If you want to wait until a treatment is "proven safe and effective" for osteoporosis, you will have to avoid all those listed above as
well as the plan in this book.

In the evidence-based paradigm, proof of the effectiveness of a treatment is based on clinical results rather than on laboratory experiments. This paradigm is the subject of the next chapter, and its happy
consequences for bones are the subject of the rest of this book.

FOUR

My Bones Are Not Your Bones:
The Clinical Nutrition Approach

CAN A NEW WAY OF THINKING lead not only to a new approach to a problem, but also to different results? Instead of assuming, for example, that all bones are the same and will be healed with the same approach for everyone, where would the premise lead that all bones are different and need different approaches to heal? In other words, what if "my bones are not your bones"?

It was this enigma that I encountered as I became acquainted with the clinical nutrition paradigm through a muscle-testing method. My local chiropractor had already figured out that my body needed calcium, and I had been taking an over-the-counter brand. But my back problems kept recurring; I'd suddenly have to call for help because I was down on the floor and couldn't move. Because of chronic deep muscle tension that kept pulling my back out of alignment, he referred me to a health practitioner skilled in body work, Laura Samartino.

Soon after she began working on this muscle tension, she began training in muscle testing and assessed me. I both dutifully and doubtfully began taking the whole food concentrates she recommended for me. My progress seemed slow, I thought, but I reminded myself not to be impatient after years of becoming increasingly decrepit, even though I wanted results yesterday.

When I heard there would be a professional training seminar in my area, I decided to attend. It would be an understatement to say that my initial experience with the clinical nutrition paradigm as contrasted with the medical one was dissonant. As a card-carrying, currently licensed, university-educated member of the modern medical system, I had cut my teeth on Western medicine. I was unaware of its underlying philosophy, nor did I begin to comprehend its implications until I discovered the contrasting clinical nutrition approach. With considerable effort, I forced my former assumptions to sit in the back of the room while I opened my mind to hear the speaker without prejudice. As I listened, it dawned on me that the ramifications of this new approach were profound. If clinical nutrition truly had the power to restore health, then the pharmacological and surgical approaches of the medical model were seriously restricted.

The analogy used to explain muscle testing is that the body is like a computer, with the brain as the memory bank and electricity generator, and the thousands of miles of nerves as the electrical wiring that connects every part of the body. The brain will compute anything if you know how to ask the question; the nerves connect with fuses or breaker switches called reflexes. Muscle testing is a way of asking the brain how its various parts are functioning.

This idea that the body has an electrical system initially seemed strange to me, but upon reflection, I realized I was taught the same thing in physics and chemistry. All matter, the body included, is made up of molecules composed of atoms, electrons, protons, and neutrons, every one of which is electrical. An electrical charge is a quantity of positive, negative, or neutral energy. In this case, it is present in a body tissue. Chemically it is referred to as valence, which is the capacity to attract, repel, or interact with magnetic forces. The instructor was harnessing this charged energy via an indicator muscle as he demonstrated how to test the state of the electrical charge of various anatomical systems.

So I stayed for the whole seminar that day as the instructor demonstrated electrical reflexes in over a hundred seminar participants and outlined the corresponding clinical nutrition protocols. And I stayed the course with my own protocols recommended by my practitioner and my teachers. I also continued seeing Laura. It had taken twenty-five years to reduce my bones to their current porous state, we reasoned, so I'd have to give this method a chance to work, as indeed it did. As I began to experience greater and greater health improvements, I became more enthusiastic and also more curious about what this method could do. I began attending classes taught by Kim Sperry, C.N.C., a nutritional specialist of considerable knowledge, to learn how to assess nutritional needs via muscle testing. Within a few years, not only did my bones recover, but I was more active, vital, alive, agile, and strong than I had been since my mid-twenties. I had also progressed sufficiently in clinical nutrition training so I could make it available to my clients.

A few years to restore complete health after twenty-five years of consistent bodily decline is not a bad bargain in my opinion. Still, why did it take so long to find help? The answer lies in how the body heals and how clinical nutrition works.

THE CLINICAL NUTRITION PARADIGM

The clinical nutrition approach assumes that each of us is biochemically unique. Even if two people with the same diagnosis are close relatives, each will require a unique healing strategy. Seven principles of clinical nutrition are significant for all bodily systems, including bone health:

- The body wants to be healthy.
- The body is made of three things—water, air, and food.

- In order to heal, the body uses food.
- The body knows how to heal and will do so if supported with the right building blocks (in the form of food).
- Bodily processes can become so unbalanced that the amount of particular nutrients found in food are insufficient to restore balance and health.
- Foods can be concentrated to clinical potency to deliver greater nutritional impact than foods normally found in nature, and targeted to particular systems (including bones) so the body can heal itself.
- Given enough time, the body will heal itself.

These principles underlie holistic health approaches. Expressions of an empiric tradition, they are not a substitute for medical assessment or standard medical care. Rather, these principles aim to balance the body and improve its vitality.

Clinical nutrition developed from healing traditions as diverse as the three-thousand-year-old Chinese practice of acupuncture and the comparatively more modern school of empiricists or vitalists, beginning in the fifteenth century. Vitalists consider attitudes, behaviors, feelings, tensions, addictions, and pains as being unique to each individual rather than applicable to all. They see these manifestations as disturbances in vitality, and rather than seeking to eliminate symptoms, they aim to improve vitality. Stimulating growth or balance of the life force through nutrition is one such way to improve vital energy.[1]

Muscle testing is a way to assess the nutritional balance that contributes to improved vital energy. There are many systems of muscle testing. The first, Applied Kinesiology, was introduced by George Goodheart, D.C., in 1964. Various other methods have been developed since that time.

THE CLINICAL NUTRITION ASSESSMENT PROCESS

All health practitioners rely on clinical experience to determine how to address their clients' needs. Some also employ a client interview or a variety of laboratory tests, which can include blood work, saliva tests, urine tests, or hair sample assessments.

Michael Dobbins, D.C., is an internationally renowned lecturer in the field of nutrition therapy and a former college professor and instructor in the U.S. Navy Nuclear Submarine Program. He teaches health professionals how to use a Symptom Survey Form to assess their clients' need for nutritional balance. Practitioners may have people fill out the Symptom Survey Form on their first visit and provide a summary report on the second visit. Muscle-testing practitioners often have clients fill out a Symptom Survey Form to identify problem areas and to develop a baseline for evaluating outcomes. In addition, they use a method of muscle pulsing and resistance to assess what the body needs to heal itself.

This use of body electricity to assess the functional state of organs operates on the same principle as the electrocardiograph or EKG machine, which records the heart's electrical energy pattern. But instead of using a machine, the muscle-testing practitioner connects directly with points on the client's skin, creating a circuit between these points and an indicator muscle. The person being tested holds out an arm, and the practitioner presses down on the test muscle while assessing each reflex in turn.

This method can yield a veritable encyclopedia of information. It can also pick up tendencies toward disease long before they would show up in laboratory tests. For example, if muscle testing demonstrates that bones have too much electricity, we know they may develop spurs. Or if muscle testing demonstrates a deficiency of omega-3 oils, practitioners may recommend sufficient oils to carry minerals to the bones. Nonetheless, Michael Dobbins, D.C., states, "Muscle testing is an art form and should be treated as such."[2]

CLINICAL NUTRITION PROTOCOLS

Once a nutritional assessment is completed, the health practitioner then designs a personalized clinical nutritional protocol that uses whole food concentrates and/or therapeutic-strength organic whole herbs. The nutritional protocols are based on formulas developed by Royal Lee, D.D.S. An inventor and electrical engineer holding over one hundred patents, including some for guidance systems used by NASA, Dr. Lee became a dentist after designing dental equipment. Seeing a major increase in dental cavities, Dr. Lee concluded that "we are dying by the mouthful." [3] To counteract this trend, he designed his first whole food concentrate, Catalyn (i.e., a nutritional "catalyst"), which people could take three times a day. (For more about Catalyn see chapter 9.) He scouted out the richest soil possible, which he found in Wisconsin—rich, alluvial soil deposited by glaciers. There he grew the ingredients for Catalyn and developed the standardized process of making whole food concentrates.

Westin Price, D.D.S., another dentist, was an associate of Dr. Lee. He studied the diets of primitive cultures around the world, where the young might die of trauma, but not because of degenerative diseases.[4] Other members of these cultures lived to very old ages, while living on nature's diet.[5] His findings were the same as Dr. Lee's: the degenerative diseases of Western civilization had everything to do with a degenerating nutritional state.

Dr. Lee, a genius and a pioneer in clinical nutrition, is often referred to as the world's greatest nutritionist. In the 1920s, he founded the Standard Process Company, which has continued to produce his formulas for pure foods concentrated to clinical potency. The company grows its organic ingredients on its own farms in rich soil that is free of soil-depleting chemical fertilizers, herbicides, and pesticides. Their products are also free of coloration and coatings, which contributes to their potency.

The potency of whole food concentrates is essential to physical healing. Mary Jane Mack, R.N., who practices in Seattle and teaches nationally, says, "I use only Standard Process products because I have predictable results. I know each month if something's not right. I know exactly what people need to do to achieve peak performance."

She adds, "I see people coming in who are on all these other products, and underlying they still have the same problem. I've been open to other products; I'm open for my clients' best interests, what's best for them, but I haven't found anything close to Standard Process. I see just about everything . . . every latest multilevel product, things other doctors and naturopaths have recommended. Some look like good products but just don't get the job done."[6]

Many non–whole food products are made of synthetic vitamins, which are like a picture or model of the real thing: they are constructed similarly but have no life in them. Real food concentrates can impart real life to the body. The radiation of this life impulse can be seen in chromatographs, which picture a substance in various colors as determined by its dominant wavelengths. As Judith DeCava, M.S., C.C.N., states, "It is simply a matter of chemistry versus biochemistry."[7]

The body does not know how to process high dosages of artificial vitamins. Many synthetic vitamins are "coal tar [or petroleum-based] reproductions of isolated chemical formulas of vitamin structures reproduced in a laboratory. They . . . also lack the synergistic elements normally present in whole foods. . . . They often make you more deficient and out of balance and can create other problems because they do not contain all the co-factors [additional nutrients and enzymes] found in nature which made the vitamins work."[8] The body has to borrow the missing nutrients and enzymes from its own nutritional stores, thus depleting the body further. Counterfeit supplements can actually pollute the body, clog the elimination system, build up in the liver, and create toxicity.

The benefit of botanical nutrients over synthetically manufactured ones has been scientifically validated as far back as 1848 by Louis Pasteur, who discovered differences in their crystalline structure and molecular configuration. For example, organic molecules are either left- or right-handed; thus, their chemical makeup may be precisely identical but their crystalline structure different. The body not only knows whether it wants a right- or left-handed molecule, it also knows which one it is receiving and whether or not it fits. But pharmaceutical manufacturing processes cannot select for one or the other.[9]

Michael Dobbins, D.C., states that "Dr. Lee concentrated food products and found out what created the greatest therapeutic change. Only later have some of the reasons why it works become apparent. One example is a vitamin which was named vitamin B_4 when it was discovered in England. However, it has never been discovered [meaning officially recognized] in the U.S." He adds, "Natural ones contain essential associated food factors in the form of enzymes and co-enzymes that are required for the full beneficial effects. Lee's products succeeded as much by their unknown factors and effects as by the ones that were known or are known. Many of the factors are still unknown."[10]

Dr. Dobbins, who teaches clinical nutrition to health professionals, points out that synthetic vitamin B_1, for example, can irritate the peripheral nerve plates and create toxic symptoms. "The body does not have the enzymatic mechanism to ingest more than five milligrams of B_1 per day—more than that results in female sterility by the second generation. The symptoms of this overdose include fast pulse, irritability, tremor, and weakness."[11]

Dr. Dobbins continues, "The issue is not the molecule, it's the package. The person who is deficient can handle the food form, but they can't handle the massive dose of a synthetic. The body has to draw from its reserves everything it needs to handle this massive dose, and therefore becomes further depleted. It taxes the patient's body far too much. The body may not know the difference in a molecule of one nutritional factor, but it knows the rest is lacking. That's why there's a rebound effect. The end result is production of deficiency states that are worse than the ones they began with."[12]

Because many health care practitioners understand the significance of using whole food concentrates, they often recommend Standard Process products. The body can substitute chemical imitations of food; however, ingesting counterfeit and imitation food and chemicals can only attempt to compensate for the real thing. Informed practitioners point out that such substitutions are dangerous because they can actually weaken the body, making it easy prey for microbes when even a slight cell malfunction occurs. The body simply cannot maintain health on food grown on depleted soil with chemical fertilizers, then adulterated with additives and sometimes contaminated with toxic substances.

Bruce West, D.C., who produces the health newsletter *Health Alert*, also recommends Standard Process's concentrated food products: "I'm talking about products that truly change your body's chemistry, allowing it to heal. These are products that alter a heart graph, dramatically reverse pathological blood tests, alter organ and gland function that is proven on objective testing. . . . The sad truth is that 95% or more of the things in your health food store and vitamin shop *cannot do this*. As such, if you are truly sick, they become a cruel hoax. There is just no way that I can recommend most of the products on the market today."[13]

He adds, "Manufacturers purport their synthetic products to be natural. . . . In the meantime, companies like Standard Process Labs continue to pay attention to the soils in its organic fields, to yield crops high in phytochemicals (whole nutrients found in plants) and to render these crops into supplements in a miraculous, patented process that maintains the integrity of the health-rendering plant chemicals . . . in over 60 years, Standard Process Labs has developed and maintained its position as the *benchmark of excellence* in the entire industry *without ever advertising at all!*"[14]

The organic whole food concentrates such as those made by Standard Process are also formulated with a different philosophy from most others. For example, their contents are designed to carry out a particular function rather than to contain a certain number of milligrams of an isolated nutrient. Standard Process states that their approach is "to give the patient the specific food factors that are lacking, along with the associated factors that make it work."[15] Thus labels may state that they contain far less of a nutrient in milligrams than manufactured vitamins. However, because that nutrient is accompanied by all the cofactors the body needs to use it, fewer milligrams are required. The converse is also true. Because manufactured vitamins are chemical imitations of food and lack the cofactors they need for proper absorption and utilization, greater milligram dosages are required to approach a beneficial effect.

Many of Standard Process's products also contain protomorphogens, or PMGs, in concentrated amounts. Protomorphogens are the biological template for organs. They are complexes made up of nucleoprotein molecules, a phosphorus backbone, and a mineral substrate with as many as sixty to ninety trace minerals. PMGs have an affinity for fibrin, which means they're attracted onto connective tissue. They provide proteins with the patterns to become bone, liver, or adrenal glands, for example. They provide the mineral substrate the DNA uses to give directions to the binding site when building body tissue such as organs, glands, or bones.

PMGs are the smallest unit of the cell blueprint assembly. They are "growth factors" because cells will fail to grow without them. Without PMGs, states Michael Dobbins, D.C., "the cell becomes senile and dies." He adds, "Some people have a failure at that level. They appear to have a genetic deficiency but it's really not. Their bodies are expressing a familial deficiency state that's been passed down for generations."[16] Protomorphogens are especially important when an organ or system is functioning less than optimally. PMGs act like a guidance system that tells nutrients to go to a particular organ to support it.

Individually designed protocols are made to be ingested daily over the length of a major healing cycle: a three-month period. Feeding the body the nutrients it needs during that three month cycle can result in a shift to regeneration from degeneration.

Because the potency of whole food concentrates is well known to the vitamin industry, some companies have recently begun to advertise products that seem like whole food concentrates. However, a careful reading of their literature demonstrates they are using synthetic vitamins: for example, one company's product literature states, "We add . . . a very small amount of the USP vitamin or mineral" to the food and bacteria, thus relying on the bacteria to somehow convert the synthetic vitamins to whole foods.

Another product is listed as "nutraceutical grade." Any product called "nutraceutical" has been chemically altered from its natural state."[17] This same company's vitamin C is one such product. According to the Food and Drug Administration's loose definition, USP grade vitamin C is just ascorbic acid, which is only one component of true vitamin C complex. Ascorbic acid is made in the laboratory by boiling corn syrup and sulfuric acid together. Since many people cannot tolerate corn, their bodies react negatively to this "vitamin C," and in some cases, it strips the lining of their intestines.

There are a few other companies that are making similar "food state" products. On investigation, however, we find that they are simply adding synthetic chemical vitamins to food, then adding bacteria and letting the bacteria digest the synthetic vitamin, and packaging the product in tablet form. But the body knows the difference. Synthetic vitamins work well for the first couple of weeks, but then the results go downhill.

In addition to whole food concentrates, clinical nutritional protocols can include therapeutic-strength organic whole herbs. In fact, sometimes whole herbs act synergistically with whole food concentrates to yield maximum therapeutic effect with fewer pills. Kerry Bone of Australia founded MediHerb in 1986 to provide such quality therapeutic-potency organic herbal extracts. An experienced research and industrial chemist, Bone graduated from the School of Phytotherapy in the United Kingdom and became a practicing herbalist. Bone created MediHerb because he wanted efficacious herbal therapy to be available instead of only poor quality extracts.[18]

MediHerb uses high-quality, carefully selected, organic whole herbs from sustainable cultivated sources. They use a unique, revolutionary method for obtaining an optimal full-spectrum extract of the original herb while preserving high levels of the known active qualities. Their extraction process uses cold percolation so no heat will destroy the delicate chemical bonds of the herbs, and each herb has its own unique percolation process to optimize it. They employ herbalists and naturopaths, all of whom continue to see patients in their clinical practice. In addition, the company works with a board of leading Australian and international herbalists to ensure that their products are effective in clinical practice. They also produce a wide range of professional publications, including research papers, clinical journals, and newsletters. (See appendix II for more on whole herbs.)

EVALUATING RESULTS

Most health care practitioners working with herbs and nutrition focus on functional outcomes, which means finding what works. Bruce West, D.C., refers to this approach as "*evidence-based medicine:* making observations to see what obviously improves the health of the patient. . . . Evidence-based medicine involves trial and error . . . finding out what solves your particular problem. . . . Keep in mind that what works for person A may fail for person B."[19]

In addition to clinical experience, health practitioners use lab tests to determine whether their recommendations were effective. Practitioners using the Symptom Survey Form detect groups of symptoms that relate to changes in the balance of particular organs, glands, or bodily systems.

Since formal research on the benefits of clinical nutrition protocols is just beginning, its success at helping people recover their bones can only be approximated as of this writing. There are currently 150,000 practitioners in the United States who use whole food concentrates. If the rate of osteoporosis is one in six people, then one in six of these practitioners' clients would likely have nutritional imbalances that correlate with bone health.

I attempted an informal survey and discovered a range of responses. Dr. Bruce West in Monterey, California, has maintained a long-standing, active, full-time practice and generates a monthly newsletter with subscribers across the United States. His approach to patients with suspected osteoporosis includes balancing their nutritional state. When asked how many patients with osteoporosis had improved bone health after treating their nutritional state, he replied, "Four to five thousand."[20]

Elaborating further, he reported, "Most patients have osteoporosis. For most who suffer an osteoporotic hip fracture, I think their hips are broken before they even fall, and that's what makes them fall. The regular pressure and tension of the muscles and ligaments is enough to fracture a bone in someone who's osteoporotic. The osteoporosis is what's making them fall down in most of the cases."[21]

Mary Jane Mack, R.N., has practiced in Seattle, Washington, for many years. She also leads her own workshops all over the country. She says she has "helped lots of people prevent osteoporosis. That's what we do all the time."[22] She estimates that over the course of her practice, she's helped maybe a hundred people who've been medically diagnosed.

Clearly, clinical nutrition protocols have saved a lot of people from tremendous suffering. Nonetheless, from a scientific point of view, such information will continue to be considered merely anecdotal until formal research is complete.

Meanwhile, from a personal point of view, these scientifically unaccounted-for people are undoubtedly grateful like I am, every day, for the powerful benefits of this healing method. They, too, must be very happy that they did not have to wait around while scientific debate took place and their health declined even further. Or perhaps they are too busy leading full and rewarding lives even to think about it.

What, then, are the essential components in the quest for perfect bones?

The Bare Bones of Healing Bones: The Six-Point Plan

THE WORKING PRINCIPLE behind the Six-Point Plan for Healthy Bones is supporting nature's built-in process for keeping bones healthy. When bones first form in the embryonic stages of life, the necessary nutrients to make them are delivered via rich maternal blood. Normal prenatal bone development depends on nutritional factors being pumped in through the baby's umbilical cord. After birth, that job falls to our own blood supply. The quality of this blood, therefore, is central to bone health.

Clinical nutritionists generally believe that nutritional poverty is at the root of osteoporosis, and that it is essential to provide nutritional enrichment to build bone. Good nutrition builds up the bone bank account. This is especially so in the second half of life because by then many of us have used up the nutritional storehouse with which we were born. If we don't actively replenish this storehouse during midlife, we can end up paying severe health penalties.

This way of thinking about bone health stands in contrast to the idea that bone health is a question of calcium intake only, or perhaps calcium and estrogen. But bones are made of far more than just calcium. They are made from vitamins, minerals, hormones, enzymes, hormone precursors, and antibodies, all in the right proportion.

Actually, calcium can fatigue the older heart if it is not combined with other foods that build the blood. When extremeties are swollen due to heart fatigue, live foods, such as those in whole food concentrates, can gradually pull water back from swollen extremities.

The protocols listed in part three outline combinations of whole food and whole herb products that build blood from living food so bones can build living tissue.

LAYERS OF HEALING

Any process of healing is composed of layers, and this is also true for healing bones. How might that process of discovering layers unfold? To see how layers play into this healing process, let's explore the case of Sophia Tampinelli, a woman concerned not only about her bone health but about her overall health.

To arrive at Sophia's house is to be welcomed with all the warmth of her Italian heritage. We first sat in her beautiful garden where the sounds of a splashing fountain and strains of opera floated on the evening breeze. Her cat soon joined us, purring contentedly. Visiting her after returning from the first clinical nutrition seminar I attended, I enthusiastically reviewed what I had discovered: "You get tested to find out what your body is saying and then follow the protocols to correct imbalances. Because the body's needs are layered, you usually come back every three months, about once each season, to see what your body needs next, if anything. And each time your body is in better health, getting more finely tuned, and constantly improving." As she had suffered recent and repeated bouts of ill health, Sophia listened intently and decided to give this clinical nutritional approach a try. After a few months, I returned to interview her and find out how things had gone.

First, we reviewed her history. An elementary school teacher, Sophia would turn fifty-five in another month, a ripe age for developing obvious osteoporosis. She reported that she was often bone tired. No bone weakness was ever medically diagnosed, yet she recounted many clues that her bones were not in the best of health: "feeling brittle, my back goes out easily, my left hip goes out, I have pain in my spine in between my shoulder blades. If I lean on my wrists too hard they hurt too." All this seemed to start, she said, around fifteen years earlier when she was forty. To address it, she took up stretching exercises and saw a chiropractor a couple times a year. She also occasionally took synthetic vitamins and minerals.

But she thinks this problem began in childhood. "I had poor teeth as a child. I relate that now to having malnourished bones. By age twenty I'd had all my teeth out. But that wasn't all. I started my period at age eight. At age twelve I had a D & C because I had a period where I hemorrhaged for forty days. I always had excessive periods. I had fibroid cysts on my ovaries, too, so my hormones might not have been working right.

"I married at eighteen, and had five miscarriages when I was eighteen, nineteen, twenty, twenty-one, and twenty-two. There were all kinds of theories about why—mostly it's God's will, or nobody knows, but nothing was ever found about why all this was happening. Besides, back then, doctors were gods and you didn't question." In her early twenties, she had a total hysterectomy. "After that I was on estrogen (Premarin) around ten years before I noticed scary warnings in the packages that said if you've taken it more than six months at a time there's an increased cancer risk. So I went off it, and have been on and off it for the last twenty years."

Then six years ago she was medically diagnosed with diverticulitis. "They took out a section of sigmoid colon and my gallbladder at the same time because I had a big stone that had bothered me for years. After surgery I gained sixty or seventy pounds and still haven't lost it all. I guess my digestion still wasn't working right."

Layer One: Bones were not Sophia's first layer of health problems. Her muscle-testing evaluation brought up the possibility of "an enlarged heart and chemical poisoning. For that I took Parotid PMG [a product designed to support the body in removing chemical poisons]" (see chapter 11).

Layer Two: After her heart was stronger, Sophia followed a protocol to support her sex hormones (see chapter 9). For this she took natural ProGest Cream, Utrophin, and a core nutrition protocol (to improve her general nutritional status): a combination of RNA, Organic Iodine, B_6 Niacinaminde, and For-Til B_{12}. She reports, "I lost twenty-four pounds in a few months. I also felt my sense of well-being return. I felt less brittle."

Layer Three: Sophia said, "We also found an indication that I needed nutrition to support gallbladder functioning, despite the fact that it had been surgically removed. This is because of a weakness in function rather than the organ itself." For this third layer, she took A-F Betafood, which helps improve the quality of bile, so essential for metabolizing the oils that carry calcium to the bones. These essential fatty acids are the precursors to every hormone in the body. "I'd always had trouble eliminating, but when I went on the A-F Betafood, that changed. I felt clean and regular, with no toxic bowel, and I was thinking better."

Layer Four: A fourth layer addressed parasites (for which she took Multizyme) and liver toxicity. "I feel we have been working on a causal chain, working backward to get to deeper and more basic problems. I'm getting a better understanding of how it all works and what I need, especially the minerals. I'm from an Italian family, and I remember drinking wine as a child, but not milk. My father was from

Italy, and he made wine." Between a pasta-rich diet and low calcium supply, it is likely that she was deficient in basic bone-building minerals during this crucial bone formation period.

Layer Five: After all the above protocols, Sophia's body indicated its readiness to heal her bones. She tested as needing two final protocols: one for pituitary support and one for bones.

Sophia's story demonstrates a basic principle of a holistic approach to health. As Jonathan Wright, M.D., of Washington's Tacoma Clinic, put it: "To take care of our bones, we must take care of our whole bodies and our overall health. What's good for the bones is good for the heart, the skin, the breasts, the stomach, and even crucial for future generations."[1]

Would Sophia's layers of protocols be right for someone else? Probably not. They were definitely different than my body indicated. Nor were they the same for Carol Gieg, whose search had taken her to eleven physicians. She discovered her own first layer when she went to Kim Sperry, C.N.C., a nutritional counselor. Unlike Sophia and me, Carol needed adrenal support initially. Her protocol included Cal-Amo, a product to acidify her body and restore mineral balance, a calcium replacer, a whole food vitamin product called Catalyn, and flax seed oil. Far from delaying her bone healing, concluding this first phase set the physical stage necessary for bone healing to occur.

Thus clinical nutrition has a double-edged health benefit. Improving the nutritional state of bones improves the health of the entire body. And addressing conditions not apparently related to bones indirectly improves bone health. Michael Dobbins, D.C., summarizes, "You provide nutritional support for a person who has a problem."[2] What, then, are the common denominators in such a healing program?

THE SIX-POINT PLAN FOR HEALTHY BONES

A truly effective program considers nutritional needs for all six points of the Plan for Healthy Bones. To review, these points are:

1. Healthy connective tissue
2. Sufficient minerals and their vitamin helpers
3. Essential fatty acids and the ability to metabolize them
4. A balanced hormonal system
5. Proper digestive, eliminative, and muscular activity
6. A clean environment and healthy immune system

Part two explores each of these points in its own separate chapter. Each point has a unique emphasis on building particular blood nutrients so blood can build bone.

The Six-Point Plan for Healthy Bones will help you understand what goes into building perfect bones. Then you are in a position to find a good practitioner and get a good evaluation. And when your health practitioner assesses your body's needs, you'll be better able to stay the course and follow the recommended protocols because you'll better understand what's involved. Your body will do the rest. General protocols are provided in the last chapter.

PART TWO

The Six-Point Plan

SIX

Building the Bank:
Healthy Connective Tissue

HARD BONE MAY SEEM to have little in common with supple ligaments, but actually they are closely related. Without healthy connective tissue, bones cannot form properly. That's because bones are constructed on a mesh of fibers made of collagen (a connective tissue). In fact, connective tissue is referred to as "osteoid," which means "bone-like." Connective tissue is the protein matrix on which bones form. "Bones can be thought of as mineralized cartilage," states John Lee, M.D.[1]

Healthy bones are not brittle or weak; they are supple and strong. Connective tissue provides the suppleness. Therefore, to be healthy, bones need healthy connective tissues.

Connective tissue is one of the four main tissues of the body. It binds together everything from the smallest cell to the largest organ. It's found everywhere in the body. It gives form to vascular tissues such as blood and lymph; its fibers make up the walls and hold the shape of all seventy-five thousand miles of blood vessels, so blood can flow through them. When a body is out of balance, connective tissues in arteries can become bony due to mineral deposits, a condition called hardening of the arteries, which contributes to dementia, strokes, and heart attacks. A new technology, electron beam-computed tomography (EBCT), can now produce computerized images of these arterial calcium deposits.

Connective tissue formed into strands that are woven together produces ligaments. Ligaments connect the ends of bones to other bones, to cartilage, or to other structures where they either facilitate or limit motion. Connective tissue supports visceral organs and keeps them in place so they don't all fall down on each other. It also sustains the shape of intervertebral discs that keep spinal bones from rubbing together and crushing delicate nerves. In addition, the fibrous network furnishes strength for skin, hair, nails, and tendons.

Connective tissue also stores food. Michael Dobbins, D.C., points out that "connective tissue holds substrates [the underlying substances acted on by enzymes] in reserve until cells need them and hormones stimulate their release."[2] Thus, connective tissue also plays a role in blood formation and in some immune defense mechanisms.

Bone-building cells turn soft, pliant connective tissues into hard, strong bones. These cells use chlorophyll and green plant material to form proteins and trace minerals to produce an organic mesh. Once formed, this flexible fibrous net holds the various minerals that form bone in rigid, crystalline structures. The particular kind of protein mesh that makes up the bone bank's safe-deposit box is called collagen.

Collagen is the foundation for bone well-being. Without it, the body would merely be a mass of parts with nothing to hold it together. Given how important connective tissue is to every part of the body, keeping it healthy pays big health dividends. Indeed, when this tissue disappears, the calcium and other bone bank mineral deposits that were bound to it go too. Without connective tissue, the mineral deposits that make up bone have nowhere to go.

Some connective tissue weaknesses make themselves known with a bang, others with a whimper. For me, it was a whimper of sorts, initially a matter of minor curiosity. Fingernails broke throughout the day. There were occasional, small skin bruises, easily dismissed in the winter. The following summer, the bruises were bigger, so people often remarked, "Wow, what happened to you?" as they pointed at a huge black-and-blue discoloration. "I don't know," I'd reply. But the bruises were so huge that I thought surely I'd remember hurting myself that badly.

Carrying the weight of a backpack with water and a few other supplies became uncomfortable. I focused on building muscle strength, but felt like my muscles were working overtime. My back seemed to slip out of alignment too easily. Late that fall, I suffered an extruded disc.

The symptoms of someone else's connective tissue weakness might not show up the same way mine did. In fact, for many it begins as something they interpret as merely cosmetic. They look in the mirror and see the "sag and bag" syndrome, or severe skin wrinkling. Uncomfortable about looking bad, some people may even seek, not better nutrition, but plastic surgery. For tennis or racquetball players, it may show up as tennis elbow. Runners may develop knee pain. People who walk or stand may develop fallen arches in their feet. Someone else may have trouble keeping their bones aligned; they pick up a bag of groceries or a briefcase and pull their shoulder out. They throw a baseball, and their elbow pops. They make a small jump and sprain their ankle.

When connective tissue is weak, muscles tighten, taking over the work that ligaments were designed to do. But when muscles work overtime and connective tissue remains unrepaired, muscles, too, will eventually fatigue. Reaching this state, organs may drop from their proper place in the body, placing strain on themselves and other organs. Kidneys can drop, putting pressure on certain muscles and immobilizing others, causing the pelvis to destabilize and the sacroiliac joints to go out of alignment. The blood vessels in the gastrointestinal tract may weaken, contributing to the development of hemorrhoids. The uterus or bladder also may drop, in severe cases leading to the recommendation of surgery to repair it. The ligamental ring that holds the stomach in place may slacken, allowing some of the stomach and its acid to burn the esophagus, a problem often referred to as acid reflux disease or a hiatal hernia. When inguinal ligament rings loosen, portions of the intestine can enter them. Such an inguinal hernia is a dangerous condition, for the intestines can strangulate.

However bone weakness makes itself evident, the relative condition of the connective tissue matrix can lead to one person suffering a fracture and another not, even though they have the same bone density. Osteoporosis and osteoarthritis are both disturbances in connective tissue, expressed in different ways.

Connective tissue weakness may be caused by a drug. For example, aspirin blocks the growth of new cartilage and accelerates joint deterioration. Collagen deficiency may be connected to an injury such as a fall. Weak connective tissue can also be caused by exercise or surgery. Being excessively over- or underweight also plays a role. Allergic reactions may weaken tissue. For many, an alkaline pH has caused connective tissues to erode. Some report that silicon breast implants started their connective tissue problems, leading to fibromyalgia, a debilitating condition characterized by extreme exhaustion, weakness, and pain.

Many other catalysts can weaken connective tissue. Heavy metal toxicity, as from mercury, is one such substance. The sun's ultraviolet rays, when they penetrate the skin's second layer, result in the skin wrinkling and aging. The body produces two toxic substances that can be of concern. One occurs when overstressed and weakened adrenal glands secrete cortisol, a substance that is toxic to connective tissue, causing it to lose strength. The other takes place when guanidine, a highly alkaline and toxic substance, is produced as a result of a toxic bowel.

However it starts, the decline of connective tissue health is like the proverbial canary in a coal mine. Because connective tissue is the base for all bones, its deteriorating health signals that bone health will also deteriorate if something isn't done. And connective tissue health is negatively affected far more easily than bone health. However it begins, doing something effective to restore connective tissue health is crucial to maintaining bone health.

THE BUILDING BLOCKS OF CONNECTIVE TISSUE

Connective tissue is built from certain essential materials, primarily protein, silicon, manganese, vitamin C complex, vitamin E complex, and vitamin A complex. Providing the body with these materials helps keep connective tissue in the best possible shape. For how to deal with toxic substances, see chapter 11.

Protein

Connective tissue mesh is made from proteins chained together. Proteins, in turn, are made up of chains of essential amino acids. Essential amino acids are heat labile (destroyed by heat), therefore a sufficient quantity of raw foods is central to the health of connective tissue.[3, 4] Connective tissue weaknesses are much more likely to develop in people whose food sources are overcooked with little raw content. Among the best food sources for essential amino acids are raw potatoes, jicama, raw mushrooms, the rinds of citrus fruits, and raw nuts, such as almonds or sunflower seeds.[5]

Silicon

This element is found in more than one-fourth of the earth's crust, usually in rocks and generally combined with other minerals. It is absolutely necessary to the health of connective tissue, yet when inhaled into the lungs, it can cause silicosis, a disease common to stonecutters. In the body, it is found in high concentrations at the calcification sites in growing bone. The collagen content of bones is diminished without enough silicon.[6] Apparently it strengthens the cross-linkage of collagen strands.[7] Silicon is concentrated in silica in the form of silicon dioxide. It is found in horsetail and oat straw. It is also present in foods containing fiber. Processed foods have much of their fiber content removed, and people with such low-fiber diets may lack sufficient silica to keep their connective tissue strong.

Manganese

This element helps prevent cardiovascular disease, maintains reproductive and nervous system health, aids in sugar metabolism, and builds muscle. And because it is an enzyme activator (helping enzymes to release their energy), it helps increase resistance to infection.

Manganese is the principle molecule around which collagen fibers organize themselves, which is why low levels are associated with abnormally formed cartilage and skeleton. Manganese not only helps strengthen spinal discs and ligaments, it is crucial for healthy bones. "If the formation of mucopolysaccharides [used in forming connective tissue] is impaired by manganese deficiency, then the process of calcification (and consequently, bone formation, remodeling, and repair) will be impaired," says Alan Gaby, M.D.[8]

Indeed, animals whose diets are deficient in manganese form defective bones. Professional basketball player Bill Walton discovered its importance when he suffered repeated fractures that failed to heal properly due to a manganese deficiency. Manganese deficiencies are common in osteoporosis sufferers. Manganese requires other cofactors, especially vitamin B_{12}. (Standard Process's Manganese B_{12} product contains both.)

Good dietary sources of manganese are found in whole-grain cereals, nuts and legumes, especially rice bran and brown rice. As some products used to help heal spinal discs contain very large amounts of manganese, they should not be taken routinely, but only in acute situations.

Vitamin C Complex

The whole complex that makes up vitamin C acts as an antioxidant that helps protect the body from free radical damage. Free radicals are electrically charged atoms that attach to body cells and eventually can destroy them. The cumulative damage of free radicals is associated with heart attacks, cancer, chronic fatigue, and a host of other diseases. Many products on the market today are called vitamin C but contain only ascorbic acid, a synthetic chemical imitation (made by boiling corn syrup and sulfuric acid together) of one factor that makes up the natural complex. The complete food complex has components such as ascorbic acid and bioflavonoids, which include rutin, hesperidin, hesperitin, eriodictyol, quercetin, and quercetrin. These bioflavonoids are sometimes referred to as vitamin P, or vascular fragility factors in food. Their deficiency can contribute to bone abnormalities because they help keep the collagen fiber network tough. As Alan Gaby, M.D., points out, "One of the actions of vitamin C on bone is to promote the formation and cross linking of some of the structural proteins found in bone."[9]

The role of the whole vitamin C complex in bone health is profound. British sailors who spent long months at sea without benefit of fresh fruits found this out. Their gums began to bleed, and their bones began to deteriorate badly—a condition called scurvy. Vitamin C complex–rich lemons (which the British call limes) corrected their condition and gave British sailors a new nickname: limey.

It is important to remember, says Michael Dobbins, D.C., that "a tablespoon of lemon juice a day cures scurvy, but massive amounts of ascorbic acid [which is missing all other parts of the complex] will not. The ascorbic acid made from synthetic chemicals also seems to interact abnormally with iron and other chemicals in your body. The end result can be genetic damage or organ damage (as in the heart)."[10] Dr. Dwyer, of the University of Southern California, Los Angeles, reported at the American Heart Association Cardiovascular Conference, that megadoses of ascorbic acid C can actually harden arteries faster than if you didn't take it at all.

Vitamin C factors are found in blackberries, blueberries, cherries, raspberries, and salmonberries.[11] Other excellent sources are in fresh citrus fruits, green tea, onions, cherries, plums, and whole grains. Herbs with high bioflavonoid content include chervil, elderberries, hawthorn berry, horsetail, rose hips, and shepherd's purse.[12]

Remember that flavonoids or bioflavonoids do not take the place of vitamin C. To be healthy, connective tissues need the whole vitamin C complex. If you're taking a product that has only vitamin C, or a product with only bioflavonoids, you're only getting part of what your connective tissue needs. Some clinicians suggest a one-to-five ratio of flavonoids to vitamin C.

Many ascorbic acid tablets are bound together with lactose (milk sugar), a significant problem for those with lactose intolerance. Unless the label specifically states "no lactose" or "milk free" or "contains no dairy," it probably does contain lactose.

Because vitamin C complex is a water-soluble vitamin, it is excreted rather than stored in the body and must be consumed daily.

Vitamin E Complex

The contents of this complex contain eight distinct molecules that fall into two major groups: the tocopherols and the tocotrienols, which are two types of several alcohols that comprise the dietary factor known as vitamin E. Within each group, there are alpha, beta, gamma, and delta forms, and each is a slightly different molecule the body requires.[13] Vitamin E strengthens blood vessels, the heart, lungs, nerves, pituitary gland, and skin. Because a deficiency is correlated with weak ligaments and flat feet, vitamin E is also considered as central to ligament health.[14]

The E complex is fat soluble. Food sources include butter, dark green vegetables, eggs, fruits, nuts, organ meats, vegetable oils, and wheat germ. Wheat germ oil, available at health food stores, is rich in vitamin E complex. However, vitamin E becomes rancid easily. When it does so, it oxidizes to transfatty acids, which are known to increase the risk of heart disease and premature death. That's why it's best to purchase small quantities more often.

Vitamin A Complex

This complex speeds wound healing, supports connective tissue in skin, protects eyes against macular degeneration, and improves night vision. It is essential for development of healthy mucous membranes because of its role in maintaining and repairing epithelial tissue. Without vitamin A, the body cannot use protein, and therefore cannot build connective tissue. According to John Courtney, it was originally named retinol "because of its influence on the development of the retina."[15]

Michael Dobbins, D.C., points out that "vitamin A sold in the store is a beta-carotene molecule that's a cheap, industrial waste product."[16] Beta-carotene is only one of many precursors that are later converted to retinol. Dobbins adds that many people, especially diabetics, can't convert beta-carotene for use in the body.

Vitamin A food sources include fish and fish liver oil; orange, green, and yellow vegetables; milk products; liver; and orange and yellow fruits. Raw butter is another excellent source. But not all sources are created equal. The vitamin A in spinach is ten times as potent as that from fish liver oil. Vitamin A is fat soluble, and therefore can be stored in fat cells and the liver. Therefore the body does not require it every day; however, because it is stored, it can build up in the body, resulting in hypervitaminosis A.

Other Nutrients

Other nutrients also play a role in creating healthy connective tissue and healthy bones. Among these is sulfur, which, according to Michael Murray, N.D., is a necessary stabilizing nutrient for "the connective tissue matrix of cartilage, tendons, and ligaments."[17] Therefore, sulfur is critical for maintaining the elasticity and flexibility of both connective tissue and fibrous cartilage. Sulfur is a component of all cells, but about half of the sulfur in the body is concentrated in the muscles, skin, and bones. It is also prevalent in keratin, the tough protein necessary for keeping hair, nails, and skin healthy.[18] If you have arthritis, your sulfur levels may be too low. Sulfur has long been known to relieve joint pain and swelling, which is why sufferers find relief through frequenting hot sulfur springs. Foods especially rich in sulfur include meats, eggs, and dairy products. Because sulfur has been depleted from our soils, supplementation may be necessary for some people.

The hormones estrogen, progesterone, and testosterone also play key roles in the health of connective tissue. They direct processes that support the skin and the mucous membranes all over the body. Therefore, maintaining proper levels of these hormones is central to collagen production and bone bank building (see chapter 9).[19]

RESTORING HEALTHY CONNECTIVE TISSUE

If the connective tissue is weak, what clinical nutrition products will strengthen it and keep it healthy? If your practitioner finds that your reflex called "master skeletal" tests weak or that you have a spinal disc in need of healing, then your connective tissue needs to be strengthened. If so, you may have ligaments, muscles, tendons, or cartilage that need to be repaired. There are good products formulated to provide the nutrients you need. Your practitioner will be able to determine which combination will comprise the best protocol for you. The following whole food concentrate and herbal products support connective tissue health.

Protocols are made from a combination of products as determined by your health practitioner. In the product descriptions below, "SP" designates Standard Process formulations, and "MH" designates those made by MediHerb. The sources for herbal information are *Principles and Practice of Phytotherapy: Modern Herbal Medicine*, by Simon Mills and Kerry Bone, and *MediHerb Innovative Herbal Solutions Product Catalog 2001*, unless otherwise noted. All products mentioned but not described here are detailed in other chapters (see index).

Whole Food Concentrates

These products are concentrated forms of some of the foods listed above. They are supplements ingested in addition to the diet to provide intensely consolidated quantities of the particular nutrients necessary to heal body tissues, organs, or systems.

Allorganic Trace Minerals-B_{12} (SP) is high in manganese and other trace minerals, including iodine. For people who are sensitive to iodine, practitioners may suggest Manganese B_{12} (SP) instead because it does not contain iodine. Both products are high in manganese, which, according to the *Standard Process Clinical Reference Guide,* is "a muscle builder, bone hardener and ligament strengthener."[20] This product is useful when the body needs rehydrating; it is especially useful in restoring moisture in nerves when someone is jittery and can't sleep at night because their body is too acidic.

Cal-Ma Plus (SP) is also used to repair connective tissue, especially spinal discs that are slipped, swollen, or bruised. It contains calcium lactate, magnesium, and a parathyroid tissue extract (see chapter 9). Many practitioners use a combination of Cal-Ma Plus and Ligaplex II for support of connective tissue.

Cataplex A-C-P (SP) supports both the production and maintenance of collagen. It contains the nutrients in Cyruta Plus (see below) along with the A and C vitamin complexes. In fact, "Cataplex" means a vitamin-mineral enzyme complex that contains a particular whole food: all the various factors needed by that particular nutrient to carry out its activity. In addition to supporting connective tissue for healthy bone, says Dan Newell, C.N., it provides the nutritional factors that "stop collagen overgrowth in such circumstances as adhesions from endometrial scarring, or after surgery." He has used it with success for people with deteriorating bones in the mouth: "A-C-P is used to get bioflavonoids in there in combination with Biost [SP, see chapter 7], which is the bone protomorphogen (the biological template composed of nucleoproteins)."[21]

If your connective tissue weakness is associated with night blindness, low resistance to infection, cystitis, or skin disorders, your practitioner may recommend Cataplex A instead of Cataplex A-C-P, because it contains more natural vitamin A than Cataplex A-C-P.

Dr. Michael Dobbins points out that Cataplex A-C-P "contains some of the best food sources for vitamin A complex . . . all the carotenoids . . . organic carrots, organic alfalfa, dried peavine juice (the single richest source of the full vitamin E complex), vitamin A esters from fish oils, nutritional yeast, rice bran extract and oat flour (the B complexes), vacuum dried adrenal, kidney, spleen, liver (for trace minerals and cofactors to sustain the health of the tissue, needed in micro amounts), mushroom powder (which contains a critical part of the vitamin C complex), and lecithin." He adds, that rather than taking large doses of synthetic vitamin A, "small amounts of the right thing are far better than massive amounts of the wrong thing."[22]

Cataplex C (SP) is a whole food vitamin C complex containing all the factors in vitamin C that preserve the complex (ascorbic acid) and the complex itself, which helps maintain vascular integrity, promotes pro-thrombin (a substance in blood that interacts with calcium salts to produce thrombin, which helps to clot blood once it is shed), increases the oxygen-carrying capacity of the blood enzymes, including tryosinase, which is rich in organic copper. Cataplex C is made from raw whole foods.

Cyruta or **Cyruta Plus** (SP) contains ingredients from the green buckwheat plant. It is recommended if vitamin C complex is the main nutritional need. It is rich in "P" factors (factors that, together, strengthen capillaries), including vitamin C, inositol (one of the components of vitamin B complex), and bioflavonoids. That's why it strengthens connective tissue. It's also used for people with high blood pressure and vascular fragility, which is why it sometimes is referred to as the "antistroke" vitamin complex. Since it contains the nutritional factors that strengthen blood vessels, it has the additional benefit of reducing migraines. It also helps the body free itself of viruses (see chapter 11). Cyruta contains many nutritional factors that support the capillaries for people who bruise easily or have "pink toothbrush," meaning their gums bleed easily.

For-Til B$_{12}$ (SP) may be recommended for low levels of vitamin E. It contains a special type of vitamin E in combination with tillandsia (commonly known as Spanish moss). It contains a high concentration of sex hormone factors (see also chapter 9).

Ligaplex I (SP) provides nutritional support to strengthen ligaments and is often recommended for people with herniated discs, flat feet, chronic low back problems, poor ligament tone, or ligament strain, or people whose backs won't hold alignment or adjustments. Ligaplex I contains a host of factors that support the ligaments, including manganese and vitamin E.

Acupuncturist and researcher Dan Newell, C.N., often recommends Ligaplex I "in acute situations for people who have herniated discs or who have high blood levels of calcium that precipitate manganese out of the muscles and ligaments. With herniated discs, they need the higher doses of manganese. It feeds the supporting structures around the discs."[23]

Ligaplex II (SP) is another nutritional supporter of ligaments. Ligaplex II contains the same components as Ligaplex I, in slightly different proportions, plus additional factors used for people with degenerated ligaments. It has less manganese concentration than Ligaplex I, and therefore is often used for people with ongoing, chronic muscle or tendon weakness that does not involve a herniated disc. Lee Vagt, D.C., advises people in acute situations to open the capsule and suck on it so the contents can be absorbed directly through the oral mucosa. He says that way it is absorbed directly into the nutrient bath (the extracellular fluid) of the body where it can be picked up (via passive diffusion) to generate new, healthy connective tissue. [24]

OPC Synergy (SP, vegetarian) is a highly effective product for strengthening connective tissue. The OPC stands for oligomeric proanthocyanidins. These magical molecules help synthesize and metabolize collagen. Technically, they are antioxidants. They stimulate collagen fibers to cross-link optimally, and they prevent excessive cross-linkage. When OPCs bind to collagen, they help to prevent the destruction of collagen by collagenase (an enzyme that breaks down collagen).[25]

Protefood (SP) is recommended when connective tissue lacks the essential amino acids, caused by eating overcooked food or being unable to completely break down and digest proteins. Health problems such as viscous blood, decreased appetite, loss of muscular tone, cold extremities, and fatigue often accompany this lack.[26] Protefood contains some protein from animal sources.

Spirulina, or blue-green algae, is a vegetarian option used to support weak ligamental and connective tissue. According to Raymond D. Schmidt, who recommends it for treatment of leprosy, it is a "rich protein source (about 60% of dry weight) as well as a source of vitamin B complex, vitamin C and numerous trace minerals, especially iron, copper and zinc. It contains long-chain unsaturated fatty acids of the beneficial omega-3 type, such as EPA and DHA. A major cell component of spirulina is a sterol called chondrillasterol, which is a precursor of cortisone, a secretion of the adrenal gland. These sterols make up about 2% of the dry weight of some algae. Preliminary tests indicate that blue-green algae support and enhance adrenal function and stimulate growth. In addition blue-green algae contain natural antibiotics and are an excellent source of healing chlorophyll."[27] As some brands of spirulina are not effective in strengthening connective tissue, be sure to have your practitioner test the product you want to use.

Lee Vagt, D.C., reports that some vegans have used sprouts in the place of spirulina. To be effective, he says, great quantities have to be chewed until they melt and turn to water in the mouth.[28] Another vegetarian alternative is a product from DC Labs called Discguard.

Wheat Germ Oil and **Wheat Germ Oil Fortified** (SP) are two cold-processed products that contain whole vitamin E from wheat berries. Vitamin E deficiency may result in laxity of connective tissue, damage to red blood cells, infertility, miscarriage, and destruction of nerves, among other problems. (See chapter 8.)

One vegetarian protocol for strengthening ligaments uses a combination of spirulina, vitamin C complex, and manganese.[29] These are available at your local health food store. In acute situations, for faster healing, practitioners may recommend holding the spirulina and manganese in the mouth to be absorbed directly into the blood stream from under the tongue.

A different approach for vegetarians uses Calcium Lactate (SP; see chapter 7), Linum B_6 (SP; see chapter 8), and Organic Minerals (SP; see chapter 8).

Herbal Products

Bilberry (MH) contains high levels of an antioxidant called anthocyanoside. Therefore it helps protect collagen from destruction by the collagenase enzyme.[30]

Garlic (SP or MH) strengthens connective tissue by virtue of its high sulfur content. Sulfur helps maintain the integrity of cartilage. In fact, the sulfur concentration in damaged cartilage is only 33 percent of the level in normal cartilage. Sulfur inhibits the enzymes that break down cartilage: collagenase, elastase, and hyaluronidase. Garlic is the most significant sulfur-containing herb.

Gotu Kola (MH) supports healthy connective tissue especially in veins, where it tones and promotes vascular integrity. It also increases the development and subsequent maintenance of blood vessels and their connective tissue. It also appears to stimulate the synthesis of (type I) collagen by fibroblasts, another type of cell that grows into connective tissue.[31, 32]

Hawthorn (MH) supports connective tissue because it is high in OPCs, as described above.[33] It stabilizes connective tissue tone.

Horsetail (MH) is a rich herbal source of silica. Therefore it promotes healthy skin and connective tissue and the normal clotting function of blood. Horsetail also contains calcium, phosphorus, iron, magnesium, manganese, potassium, selenium, and zinc—minerals that further aid bone health. (See chapter 7.)

Nettle Leaf (MH) is another rich herbal source of silica, which stimulates chondroblasts (the early-stage cells that form collagen) to deposit keratin sulfate (a protein found in hair and nails) onto the cartilage matrix, which has to form before minerals can be deposited on it to make bone. Nettle leaf also contains minerals essential to bone, including calcium, boron, fluorine, iron, potassium, folic acid, and vitamin K. Additionally, it is a strong anti-inflammatory.

Vitanox (MH) is an herbal combination antioxidant product that contains grape seed extract, green tea, rosemary, and turmeric, delivering both lipid- and water-soluble antioxidant protection to connective and other tissues. It is high in two types of antioxidants: catechins and OPCs.[34]

Sometimes weak ligaments are due to adrenal stress (see chapter 9 for those products) or various toxins (see chapter 11). However it is strengthened, once the sturdy connective tissue mesh is in place, those flexible tissues are ready to receive rich mineral deposits that will create strong, hard, solid bone—the second component of the six-point plan.

SEVEN

Making Abundant Deposits: Sun, Bones, and Stones

NOW THAT THE CONNECTIVE TISSUE WEB for living bone is woven, the bone bank is ready to open for business and fill these supple collagen safe-deposit boxes with mineral treasure. This magical transformation is one that science calls "osteogenesis": forming and growing bone from connective tissue. Two types of nutrients take center stage in this process. The starring role goes to minerals, while the supportive cast is made up of vitamins.

To make bone deposits, minerals must enter the bone bank and then become anchored there, where they will form beautiful crystals (a form of hydroxyapatite). But minerals have many other places to go besides bones. In fact, minerals constantly move as part of a continuous cycle of regeneration. They travel from food to blood to bone to lymph to kidney and finally to urine, to be excreted. To get them to enter the bone bank and stay there, magnetic vitamins first attract minerals, then carry them into the bone bank and secure them. In this way, the entire bony skeleton repairs itself with fresh calcium and other mineral atoms, with the result that, according to Clare Dover, "adults typically replace their entire skeleton every seven to ten years" and "children replace their entire skeletons once every two years."[1]

One reason that minerals continually shift around is that they are called into service to keep the right acid-base balance for the body—essentially in the neutral range. The right acid-base balance, or pH, takes priority over strong bones, because bodily processes cannot function properly in an environment that's too acidic or too alkaline. In its early stages, a pH imbalance can cause cells to clump. Such lumps of cells can clog arteries and veins, setting the stage for heart attacks and strokes. A severe enough pH imbalance can cause death. To quickly rebalance pH, the body makes emergency withdrawals of alkaline minerals from its crystal bone bank deposits.

Many authors have linked a diet high in meat consumption with osteoporosis, assuming, therefore, that a high-protein diet leaches calcium. This conclusion seemed even more likely after an Inuit Eskimo study, in which scientists noticed that a particular tribe had both high protein consumption and a higher-than-average rate of osteoporosis. However, as Michael Dobbins, D.C., points out, "The Eskimos had a higher than normal incidence of osteoporosis, but no causal link [between high protein and bone loss] was shown."[2]

Perhaps a high-protein diet and an absence of dietary factors that can rebalance pH within the normal range is what leaches bone. Indeed, consuming a highly acid-forming diet such as one composed largely of meat, fish, and eggs without enough alkaline foods for rebalancing could leach calcium out of the bones and make them porous.

If the pH of bodily fluids is too alkaline, on the other hand, the body rebalances by rapidly drawing calcium out of blood and hiding it where it doesn't belong. The calcium thus taken out of circulation can form kidney stones and harden arteries. That's why it's unhealthy to habitually consume milk of magnesia or sodium bicarbonate; they create and aggravate an alkaline pH. Deposits of calcium into soft tissues can also be precipitated by a deficiency of phosphorus. Most fruits and vegetables yield an alkaline ash when metabolized and thus don't deplete calcium stores. Whichever way the body is out of balance, it is likely to retain water and to become bloated or swollen.

You can test your own body's pH by purchasing strips of testing paper in most pharmacies. Be sure to follow the directions on the package, and compare the results to the normal pH value for the bodily fluid you tested, i.e., urine or saliva. Remember, the lower the pH number, the higher the acidity.

Another reason that minerals keep moving in and out of bone is that muscles require calcium to contract and magnesium to relax. The most important muscle of all is the heart. Keeping it beating is critical for life to continue, which is why the heart gets priority for calcium and magnesium over any other muscle or bone. That's why the demineralization that makes bones unhealthy, if not corrected, can be followed by the loss of heart health. Fortunately, the converse is also true: improving bone health can precede improving heart health.

Luckily, the body gives earlier clues than heart failure that the vitamins and minerals needed to crystallize bone are busy elsewhere, out of balance with each other, or otherwise absent. Symptoms of vitamin and mineral imbalances are not superficial; they are early signals that a process is underway that can lead first to porous bones, then to a malfunctioning heart, and ultimately, to death. The list of warning signs at the end of chapter 1 details these clues (see pages 11 to 15).

When a serious decline in bone health due to mineral and vitamin imbalance has begun, reversing it can be a dramatic process. Such was definitely the case when my own body began to receive nutrients in the right proportion. I had already been taking over-the-counter calcium supplements with minimal benefit. When I switched to Calcium Lactate (SP; see below), I could feel my strength returning and my muscles relaxing by the hour. But that was my story; I wanted to know other stories. Renée Freeman, the caretaker of a woman with a similar experience, generously recounted one:

I take care of Berle Johns, who is eighty-three, and her husband. They've been married fifty-one years. I do all their cooking and cleaning and taking them to the doctor. Anything that happens for them, I do. Berle had polio as a child and has a dwarfed foot, so she's always walked with a limp. But she was in a wheelchair when I started taking care of her because she'd broken her other ankle. Then in January she got a compression fracture in her back from simply bending over. If just bending over fractures your back, something is wrong.

I took her to a nurse practitioner here in town, who ordered a complete body X-ray. Berle was in real pain during the test. The technician who took the X-ray said she'd never seen such thin bones. The doctor prescribed Vicodin [a painkiller] for her. Here was a woman who wouldn't even take an aspirin when she had her breast removed for cancer. Yet she was taking this Vicodin like candy. After three months the doctor said she had to get off this.

Late February I asked Kim Sperry [a nutritional specialist] if she had anything that would build bones, and she did. But Berle didn't want to do anything, so I said to her, "if you don't get up out of this bed and make an effort to turn this around I can't take care of you!" I'm sixty years old myself. I said, "Berle, you're going to have to pay for this medicine, Medicare won't pay for it." She has a doll collection, well over a hundred dolls. She was buying a doll every two months, so she quit buying dolls to pay for the medicine.

So I got this natural stuff for her. She took Calcifood Wafers [SP]. Then she also took Biost [SP] for six months. I would say within two weeks' time the pain was gone and she wasn't taking any more pain pills at all. She was getting up on her own; I didn't have to lift her or help her in any way, where before I had to help her do everything. Before you knew it, this woman was up cleaning out cupboards, doing the dishes.

Her personality changed too. She was much more open, and she was dressed when I got there. She's got 150 cardboard boxes of stuff that's brand new and never even been used. I'd had to go through all the boxes because the cat would spray them. Now Berle's gone through the whole kitchen, cleaned out every cupboard. And she's not yelling at her husband so much anymore, where before it was constant. I was like a referee. She used to scream at him like you would not believe. One day I went down there, and her husband had thrown a breadboard at her and hit her at the chest. I said, why did you do that, and he said, because she'd thrown a glass of water in his face! She's a changed person.

Before she had this fracture, Berle did nothing but sit on the couch and watch TV, not even combing her own hair or tending to her own needs. Now she's up at 6 A.M., brushing her teeth and combing her hair. She's moving around, getting exercise too. The last time we went to town, she didn't even use her walker! When you're around someone for several years and see how they are and then see the change, it's amazing. She marked down every time she took her bone stuff. She's got everything documented; she always wrote it down. She still has Vicodin pills, but she doesn't take them.

She's just taking a minimum dosage of this stuff now. She has not had any side effects. She's not taking any pain medications. She hasn't been to the doctor since January [six months ago]. It's unreal. She does hang on to furniture when she's walking because she has this terrible withered foot. Now I want to see if her nurse practitioner will do a full body X-ray to compare [the state of her bone health now].

I have sent some of this bone stuff back to my husband's sister, who's a nurse and is also ailing. Her condition is so bad she's on disability. She said she couldn't take the stuff because it smells like something dead. I said, well, if you want to continue being on Vicodin and walking around like a zombie, you can just send it back, and I'll give it to Berle!

MAGICAL MINERALS

How could such a spectacular turnaround occur in such a short time? The two supplements that Berle took were loaded with the mineral and vitamin helpers that bones need. Such minerals make up a large percentage of the body. What exactly are these substances, whose deficiency could contribute to a debility as severe as Berle's, and whose presence can lead to such a dramatic recovery?

Technically speaking, minerals are a class of substances that occur in nature. They make up inorganic substances such as quartz, feldspar, and marble. They're also found in rocks, asphalt, and coal. Minerals have a definite chemical composition and a distinct crystalline structure like those found in gemstones. Plants take these inorganic substances from the soil and convert them into organic forms, making them available for the crucial functions they perform in our bodies.

Eating a diet high in uncooked plant mineral sources is the best way to take in minerals. Raw plants contain both minerals and vitamins that are readily bioavailable, whereas cooking these green food sources, as Dr. Royal Lee emphasized, makes them relatively useless nutritionally.

The following list contains some of the essential mineral gems that make up bone bank deposits and also describes some other functions they perform. Remember that it's not your job to figure out which ones you need and in what ratio. Nature has already done that for you, so if you eat a balanced diet and avoid mineral leachers (see chapter 11), you'll easily keep a proper vitamin and mineral balance. If your body has low enough levels to require additional support, like Berle's apparently did, your practitioner can recommend supplements.

Calcium

Calcium is a major mineral player in bone health, which is why it has received a lot of attention. In nature, calcium is found combined in materials such as limestone, coal, chalk, or gypsum. In bodies, 99 percent of calcium is combined in bones and teeth. "However, the remainder, a scant 1 percent . . . circulates in the soft body tissues and fluids. Here it is used for normal bone and tooth development, blood clotting, enzymatic action and the regulation of fluid passage through the walls of tissues and cells," according to *Healthy Cell News*.[3] Calcium also plays a key role in helping nerves tell muscles when to contract, and it smoothes the flow of impulses between the brain and nerve cells.

Calcium can lower cholesterol quickly; its administration has been demonstrated to decrease cholesterol by as much as 25 percent over time (how much time is variable, but its actions begin immediately upon digesting it). Low blood calcium levels can result in low blood pressure, for the muscles that surround the arteries won't have enough calcium to contract. If calcium levels in tissues are too low, the skin may itch and even develop welts, especially when exposed to the sun. Getting sufficient calcium to the tissues can clear up the welts. It can also clear up viral canker sores inside the mouth. When sufficient calcium is available, viruses cannot enter cells to replicate.[4] Indeed, calcium is the fuel that runs the immune system. When immune cells need to immobilize an invader (a process called phagocytosis), their cells push out little ladders; these ladders are crystalline based and require calcium.[5]

Calcium administration can relieve back and neck spasms, menstrual cramps, and even labor pains. In fact, administering calcium to one expectant mother I know helped her avoid having a C-section, which she'd been told she'd require. Because her blood pressure was too high, doctors were afraid that she'd have a stroke during the muscular efforts of labor. Her labor coach provided her with a calcium-rich protocol, which she took every hour until her blood pressure came down, followed by a lower maintenance dose. Her blood pressure came down to normal, she delivered her baby girl normally, and the C-section proved unnecessary. Calcium helps muscles do their work of contracting and relaxing, which is exactly what childbirth is all about. No doubt many women go into labor already in a calcium deficit and then suffer great pain, even stalled labor, when their muscles run out of calcium stores.

Before childbirth, calcium plays a critical role in the health of pregnant mothers and their developing fetuses. Studies have shown that women who consume calcium during pregnancy can reduce the risk of pregnancy-induced hypertension and preeclampsia by as much as 70 percent.

That's not all that calcium does. It helps coagulate blood, another critical factor in childbirth, but important even if you cut your skin or bump into something. Without sufficient calcium, a minor bump can turn into a major bruise. Calcium also helps nerves transmit their impulses. This may not sound terribly important until you think about what would happen if the nerve fibers in your heart lacked sufficient calcium to fire, or your heart muscle were too deficient in calcium to relax and contract. No doubt a great many heart arrhythmias and

congestive heart failure problems begin and end with a lack of sufficient calcium.

These are a few of the reasons that, when body fluids lack sufficient calcium, they'll take it wherever they can get it. If sufficiently
challenged, the body embezzles its own mineral treasure from teeth
and bone bank deposits to support other systems more important to
survival. This fact demonstrates the true nature of osteoporosis: it is a
compensatory adaptation designed to maintain and preserve life. Demineralizing bones is a way to keep the metabolic furnaces running
and the heart beating. To the body's way of thinking, porous is better
than dead.

Bruce West, D.C., summarized some of the common nuisance and
moderately serious disease states related to the way the body uses calcium. His list includes "canker sores, herpes, shingles, kidney stones,
sensitive gums and teeth, inability to handle heat, sunstroke, fevers,
convulsions, certain types of heart arrhythmias, cramps, leg pains, and
more."[6]

With calcium so essential to life, it is indeed shocking that, according to Sharon Bortz, M.S., R.D., "80% of women and 60% of men over
35 do not get adequate calcium in their diet."[7] Formerly, research to
determine calcium need was carried out with college graduate stu-
dents. New research conducted on senior citizens has demonstrated
differing needs based on age, and the USDA Human Nutrition
Research Center on Aging recently increased recommended daily
allowances for calcium.

But where to find calcium? Calcium-rich foods include dairy foods,
asparagus, cauliflower, clams, beets, cabbage, carrots, celery, goat milk
and cheese, onions, pumpkin seeds, turnip tops, kohlrabi, raspberry
leaves, spinach, almonds, mustard greens, pinto beans, broccoli, and
tofu.[8] Additionally, because of public awareness about the need for calcium, some foods such as orange juice are being fortified with calcium.

Antacids have recently been touted as an excellent calcium source, but there are problems with this idea. For one, the calcium contained in antacids has a low bioavailability, meaning it's in a form that the body has difficulty even accessing, let alone metabolizing. Two, proper calcium absorption requires an acid stomach environment, and antacids exist to absorb that acid (see also chapter 10).

Some researchers have estimated that perhaps only 10 percent of the calcium that people ingest through diet or over-the-counter supplements is absorbable. In fact, a recent study examined whether or not increasing milk consumption protected against osteoporosis. The study population was vast: 645,221 person-years of follow up. It failed to show protective effects of dairy against osteoporosis.[9] Perhaps this is due to a problem that nutritionist Royal Lee, D.D.S., pointed out as far back as 1955. He said that, as soon as it is drawn from the cow, milk is an unstable product because it is in contact with oxygen. He explained that once in contact with air, the milk sugar (lactose) reacts with certain amino acids in the milk protein, causing these proteins progressively to disappear. Those amino acids (particularly tryptophan and lysine) are the ones that are required to build tooth and bone. Pasteurization, he added, completes this reaction so that the milk is totally incapable of rebuilding or maintaining bones and teeth.[10]

What about over-the-counter products? Again, the problem is bioavailability and ease of metabolism. According to James Balch, M.D., and Phyllis Balch, C.N.C., "Minerals cannot be turned into tablets in their pure state [because they are chemically unstable]; they must be combined with some other substance or substances to make a stable compound."[11] This often renders them bio*un*available.

The USDA recommended dosages for daily calcium intake are significantly higher than the calcium-milligram dosages in the products that Berle took, yet she recovered rapidly. The same was true for me. I took enough Calcium Lactate (SP) to give me only 250 milligrams of calcium and 50 milligrams of magnesium from that source, yet my bones grew stronger. These experiences point to the power of whole food concentrates. All the calcium in Calcium Lactate, Calcifood, and Biost is absorbable and assimilable. Therefore my body and Berle's could use everything in the concentrates. This was true for Berle despite the fact that, given her age (eighty-three), she probably suffered from low stomach-acid production, which would reduce her ability to absorb supplements with a high milligram content of calcium.

Calcium intake is definitely important, but so is avoiding calcium loss once it's ingested. That means abstaining from substances that stimulate its loss. Such substances include alcohol, salt, sugar, caffeine, highly processed foods, phosphate-rich drinks such as colas, and a diet high in acid-forming foods, such as those containing excess animal protein.[12]

But is calcium always beneficial? In a word, no. Calcium that's ingested but not absorbed can be harmful. If you don't have enough acid in your stomach, your body will be unable to absorb it. Also, if you take calcium in the absence of magnesium, most of it will go straight through your body without benefit. And that's if you're lucky. If your system is unable to eliminate it completely, the calcium you did not absorb can form stones that are stored in the gall bladder, kidneys, or urinary bladder, causing excruciating pain. Addressing these symptoms medically involves uncomfortable tests and surgery to remove the stones. (For how to address them nutritionally, see chapter 9.)

When stored in the walls of arteries, calcium hardens them (arteriosclerosis); when deposited in the vibrating membrane in ears, it can make people hard of hearing. Calcium can also calcify the heart valve. Clearly, the body makes no guarantees that it will deposit excess calcium where it can easily be removed, by the surgeon's knife or otherwise. A better option is to consume bioavailable forms in a high stomach acid environment. Symptoms similar to those of metal toxic-ity can result from too great an intake of calcium or other minerals; these can include gingivitis, tremors, mental disturbances, and kidney damage.

As studies have shown, supplementation with calcium alone has had absolutely no impact on osteoporosis. Calcium cannot do the job alone, without other minerals and vitamins necessary for healthy bones. According to Alan Gaby, M.D., "Calcium is just one of many nutrients involved in the prevention and treatment of osteoporosis . . . bone tissue is complex, dynamic, and alive and, like other tissues in the body, has a wide range of nutritional needs."[13]

Magnesium

Magnesium is what makes fireworks burn and flashbulbs pop. Taken into the body, it is both an antacid and a laxative. In addition to being a component of bone, it also converts vitamin D to its active form, D_3.[14] Magnesium is also necessary to help muscles relax, including those of the heart. It is sometimes used for nutritional support for patients with mitral valve prolapse, as people with this diagnosis often have low magnesium levels.

On a daily basis, magnesium is essential for keeping bones healthy. In fact, some sources say the real problem in osteoporosis is a lack of magnesium, not of calcium. For example, when several hundred women were given a reversed calcium-to-magnesium formula, their bone density increased by an average of 11 percent. That's a decade worth of bone loss recovered, assuming a loss of 1 percent a year in postmenopausal women.[15] You can ask your practitioner to check whether that's true for you.

Low magnesium levels are associated with porous bones, and, as studies in the United States and Europe have shown, with developing arteriosclerosis and heart attacks, heart arrhythmias (irregular beats), high blood pressure, and high cholesterol.[16] Indeed, magnesium plays a central role in keeping arteries strong. That's why health practitioners often recommend it for restoring strength to the coronary and other arteries.

Research has shown that women's ability to absorb magnesium can drop so much that by age seventy, we absorb only two-thirds as much as we did at thirty. One laboratory reports that most women over forty test low for magnesium, a problem only intensified for those who eat poorly, drink alcohol or smoke, and take diuretics or anticholinergics.[17] Stress, too, plays a central role in how much magnesium is available to the bones. When the adrenal glands put out adrenaline, they stimulate magnesium to be withdrawn from the bone bank.

As much as half of the body's magnesium is found in bones. Alan Gaby, M.D., states that a "lack of magnesium is associated with abnormal calcium crystals in the bones, and normal levels of magnesium are associated with normal crystals."[18]

Dr. Gaby points out that its deficiency can also "cause various abnormalities of calcium metabolism, resulting in the formation of calcium deposits in places where calcium does not belong."[19] There are various opinions on what the proper calcium-to-magnesium ratio should be. Standard Process's Calcium Lactate product is based on a five-to-one ratio of calcium to magnesium.

Finding the proper calcium-magnesium balance is important for bone health because too little magnesium can cause calcium to be excreted without being absorbed. Under this circumstance, the body extracts calcium from the bone bank for other needs, thus demineralizing the bones. Without magnesium, the body also cannot metabolize such essential nutrients as phosphorus, sodium, potassium, and vitamin C. Nor can it make crucial life-giving enzymes. On the other hand, too much magnesium can prevent any calcium consumed from being absorbed.

The right calcium-magnesium balance is important to heart health too. Calcium is necessary for the heart muscle to contract, whereas magnesium is required for relaxation between beats.

Naturally, each body requires a different balance, which is why nutritional protocols are individualized. Dietary sources of magnesium include whole grains, especially barley; legumes; beans; and fresh vegetables such as chard, cress, corn, peas, parsnips, green cabbage, brussels sprouts, endive, alfalfa, and watercress.[20] Current USDA guidelines recommend a daily intake of 420 milligrams for men and 320 milligrams for women.

Phosphorus

As important to bone health as calcium, phosphorus has received much less attention. It's an element that is luminous in the dark. It's also flammable, which is why it's used to make matches. If the body lacks phosphorus, high tartar levels on the teeth and gums are likely to develop.

But phosphorus must exist in the right ratio to calcium. If there's too much calcium, the teeth can erode—a systemic cause of dental cavities. John Courtney of Standard Process states, "Sometimes looking at animals gives you a clue about people. For example, take pigs fattened on grain. Grain is high in phosphorus. When pigs are young, usually about six months old, their teeth start to erode away because they are getting too much phosphorus and too little potassium and calcium."[21]

Some sources say the optimum ratio of phosphorus to calcium is one to one. Other sources say the ratio needs to be 2.5 calcium to one phosphorus. After a significant amount of research, Standard Process arrived at a normal blood ratio of four parts phosphorus to ten parts calcium. That ratio keeps calcium in liquid form in the blood so it is available to be delivered to the bone bank.[22] When the body lacks sufficient phosphorus, it deposits calcium in tissues.

Phosphorus and calcium are opposites that balance each other. Phosphorus holds calcium in solution in the body tissues during that phase of absorption in which bone bank mineral deposits are being delivered or withdrawn from bone. Thus phosphorus can actually prevent calcium from being absorbed if too much is ingested. That's one reason why drinking sodas is not healthy for bones; the phosphates in sodas compete with calcium. Likewise, too little phosphorus prevents the body from being able to use calcium, no matter how high the calcium blood levels.

John Courtney provided an example of how these two minerals affect the body. He said that cattle raised in Wisconsin are big, easygoing, and relaxed because they eat grass high in the alkaline ash minerals, especially potassium and calcium. However, in Kentucky, where there are high phosphorus and low calcium levels in the soil, breeders raise racehorses, not contented cattle. These animals are nervous and jumpy from eating grass high in phosphorus. They are loaded with energy and can't relax. Those same horses, when brought to Wisconsin, however, quiet down. The same is true of people, he says. If they're nervous and jumpy, they need calcium. If they have no energy and are fatigued and worn-out all the time, they may need phosphorus.[23] Phosphorus is found in many foods, including nuts, dairy products, corn, eggs, fish, dried fruit, and whole grains.

Iron

Iron promotes bone health, especially through its role in respiration—providing the oxygen necessary for the metabolic fires to burn brightly enough to transform food into muscle and bone. Iron is the mineral that carries oxygen in the hemoglobin molecule; without it, the body would suffocate for lack of oxygen. Iron is a mineral competitor with calcium, however, so when iron is needed for supplementation, it is best taken separately from calcium.

Trace Minerals

In addition to the major mineral players, healthy bones need small amounts of a variety of trace minerals. These include boron, zinc, copper, and strontium, among others. In a two-year clinical study, postmenopausal women who received calcium supplements in combination with zinc, copper, and manganese demonstrated a gain in bone mineral density. However, those taking calcium alone or a placebo showed increasingly greater losses. Perhaps this is because of the crucial role these minerals play in the hormone cascade that directs bone bank activity (see chapter 9).[24]

Boron. This mineral may help the body retain and absorb its bone-building minerals. A recent study involved women age forty-eight to eighty-three taking 3 milligrams of boron a day. According to William Campbell Douglass, M.D., "The boron reduced their bodies' loss of both calcium and magnesium . . . and the women taking boron actually saw a marked increase in their blood estrogen levels."[25] Their levels of testosterone also doubled (see chapter 9).

Apparently boron reduces the loss of calcium and magnesium as well as increasing estrogen levels. Studies have shown that when women have adequate boron levels, they can produce estradiol (one of the forms of estrogen) levels equal to those of women on estrogen supplementation.[26] Boron plays a key role in the body being able to make both estrogen and testosterone.

Food sources containing boron include apples, raisins, grapes, pears, legumes, leafy green vegetables, nuts, and grains.[27]

Zinc. Adequate zinc is essential to bone health because zinc helps bone cells (osteoblasts and osteoclasts) do their jobs. Without zinc, neither kind of cell could form, let alone work. Zinc, says Alan Gaby, M.D., "further enhances the biochemical actions of vitamin D . . . and the synthesis of various proteins found in bone tissue. Zinc levels were found to be low in the serum and bone of elderly individuals with osteoporosis."[28]

Zinc is also essential in activating the digestive process (see chapter 10). Zinc is a central ingredient in many enzymes that carry out thousands of different functions from cell growth to testosterone production. It also activates and boosts the body's ability to pick up nutrients in the gut and deliver them where the body needs them to be. The role zinc plays is so great that, when the body is deficient, other organs and systems deteriorate rapidly. These areas include the brain, pancreas, liver, eyes, prostate gland, and nails. Some three hundred enzyme systems cannot proceed without zinc, including protein synthesis, vitamin D uptake, DNA synthesis, cell division, body growth, sugar metabolism, calcium metabolism, and skin, brain, and stomach regulatory functions.

Unfortunately for our health, zinc is easily replaced in the body by cadmium, a toxic heavy metal found in softened water, white flour, cigarette smoke, and galvanized pipes in the presence of acidic water.[29]

Dietary sources for zinc include oysters, beets, broccoli, wheat germ and bran, milk, egg yolks, peas, beans, cress, liver, dandelion, lentils, seeds, spinach, fish, red lettuce, apples, cabbage, and nuts.[30]

Copper. This mineral "plays a role in the formation of connective tissue," states Dr. Gaby,[31] and helps to repair bone cells. So important is copper to bone health that horses grazing in the copper-deficient Florida Everglades become unusually susceptible to bone fractures, a condition corrected when copper is added to their diet.[32] Dietary sources include mushrooms, peas, leafy vegetables, seafood, red and black currants, whole grains, nuts, organ meats, eggs, poultry, and legumes.[33]

Strontium. This element's compounds resemble calcium, which is why it can displace calcium in some processes. Like magnesium, it is used in fireworks and flares. Unlike its harmful radioisotope, strontium 90, it is nontoxic and contributes to bodily health. According to Dr. Gaby, "The human body contains about 320 mg of strontium, nearly all of which is in bone and connective tissue. . . . Specifically, strontium is capable of replacing a small proportion of the calcium in hydroxyapatite crystals of calcified tissues, such as bones and teeth . . . [it] appears to impart additional strength to these tissues, making them more resistant to resorption . . . [and] appears to draw extra calcium into bones." He adds that its administration helps gradually eliminate any radioactive strontium.[34]

Manganese and silicon, two other trace minerals, were covered in chapter 6.

VITAMINS: THE MINERAL HELPERS

Vitamins activate every biochemical process. Without the help of certain vitamins, minerals cannot get into bones to strengthen them. Certain key vitamins bind minerals to each other and to the connective tissue mesh upon which bones form. Therefore these vitamins are essential to bone health. Two of the most important vitamins needed to deposit minerals into the bone bank are vitamin D and vitamin K.

Vitamin D

Vitamin D is essential for overall good health, and deficiency creates serious bone health risks. A severe vitamin D deficiency leads to a disease called rickets, which inhibits bones from developing properly. Vitamin D provides the first phase of the courier service for minerals, carrying calcium and phosphorus from the intestine or reabsorbing phosphorus in the kidney. Vitamin D carries these mineral treasures into the blood, which delivers them to the tissues or the bone bank.

Vitamin D is made naturally by our skin. When we're exposed to the ultraviolet rays of the sun, cholesterol within the skin is converted to vitamin D.[35] Glenn Miller, M.D., points out that "an area of skin six inches square exposed to the sun for about one hour every day provides the minimum daily requirement of Vitamin D."[36] Ten to fifteen minutes of sun exposure per day is usually enough sunlight for the body to be able to manufacture sufficient vitamin D. However, people who live in cold, cloudy climates where this is impossible may need to take Vitamin D during the winter months.

Some experts are concerned that people with darker skins who live in northern climates and people who take the anticancer message too far and use total sun block creams may be falling short on their vitamin D. In the first case, skin pigmentation acts as a barrier; in the second, the sun block does. A recent study concluded just that: sunscreens can lead to serious vitamin D deficiency. Researchers also discovered that the vitamin D content in milk is erratic. Many samples of milk advertised as containing vitamin D actually had none. Lack of vitamin D is associated with colon cancer, and is implicated in breast, ovarian, and prostate cancer as well as in osteoporosis and hip fractures.[37] One large dose of six hundred thousand units of vitamin D "can cure convulsions and helps cure rickets," according to *Taber's Cyclopedic Medical Dictionary.*[38] Since the body makes vitamin D naturally from cholesterol, overly low levels of cholesterol can contribute to vitamin D deficiency.

Too much vitamin D, called hypervitaminosis D, however, is harmful. High vitamin D levels can actually cause bone loss by leaking calcium from bones back into tissues. In a deficiency of its antagonists, which are contained in polyunsaturated fatty acids (see chapter 8), vitamin D takes calcium out of the bone bank and returns it to the blood, thus contributing to the development of osteoporosis. People taking a variety of over-the-counter supplements might actually develop this problem without knowing it, for vitamin D is added to many products but not necessarily listed on the label. Vitamin F (see chapter 8), the natural antagonist to vitamin D, can help counter this. With sufficient vitamin F present, the body will naturally balance production of vitamin D so as not to produce an overload.

Likewise, too much calcium can have a negative effect on vitamin D. Dr. Hector DeLuca, who has been researching vitamin D, says, "When large amounts of calcium are administered, your body turns off its production of the important vitamin D hormone, stopping the bone-remodeling process. This results in an unhealthy skeleton."[39]

The kidneys convert vitamin D to the form needed for calcium absorption. Therefore, if the kidneys aren't working properly, they can spill excessive amounts of calcium. That means potential bone bank deposits are lost. (See chapter 10, regarding proper absorption.)

Good dietary sources of vitamin D include egg yolks, cod liver oil, salmon and cod livers, and butter fat. Bruce West, D.C., recommends raw butter as an excellent source of vitamin D for women who are prone to osteoporosis, skin problems, keratotic lesions, or even skin cancer. He reports that the form of vitamin D in raw butter is a hundred times more effective than commercial vitamin D (viosterol).[40]

Milk fortified with vitamin D is another source. Still, according to the *Journal of Biological Chemistry*, as studies completed as far back as the 1930s point out, natural vitamin D is "about 100 times more potent" than any synthetic version.[41]

Vitamin K

This group of compounds is often thought of as the clotting vitamins. They also contribute to bone health by attracting calcium to the bone bank and binding it there in its crystal form. According to James Balch,

M.D., and Phyllis Balch, C.N.C., it is "essential for bone formation and repair; it is necessary for the synthesis of osteocalcin, the protein in bone tissue on which calcium crystallizes."[42] "Without adequate vitamin K," emphasizes Dr. Alan Gaby, "bones would lack structure and order and would, like chalk, be fragile and easily broken."[43] It's possible that postmenopausal women, the greatest risk group for the onset of osteoporosis, have an increased need for vitamin K in their diet.

The two main causes of vitamin K deficiency are inadequate dietary intake of it or antagonism of vitamin K by drugs. Bruising easily and bleeding from the mucosa are early signs of this deficiency, as is blood oozing from puncture sites or incisions.

Vitamin K is found in fats, fish meal, asparagus, blackstrap molasses, broccoli, brussels sprouts, cabbage, cauliflower, dark green leafy vegetables (such as kale, turnip greens, spinach, and watercress), egg yolks, liver, green peas, green beans, oatmeal, oats, rye, safflower oil, soybeans, and whole wheat.[44] Good herbal sources include alfalfa, green tea, kelp, nettle, oat straw, and shepherd's purse.[45]

Vitamin K is also synthesized by the benevolent bacteria that inhabit the intestines. As antibiotics kill these friendly bugs, it's important to bone health to replace them, both during and following a course of antibiotics. It is a much less risky and healthier option to replace intestinal flora than it is to take vitamin K unless other symptoms are present. These healthy bugs are available in capsule or liquid form in health food stores, and can also be found in yogurts containing live culture. Labels often denote live lactobacillus or acidophilus culture.

One of Vitamin K's isolates (phylloquinone, vitamin K_1) is not toxic at five hundred times its recommended daily allowance (0.5 milligram/kilogram/day). However, menadione, a vitamin K precursor, has a finite toxicity, or time limitation, depending on the availability of sulfhydryl groups with which it can interact; it can cause hemolytic anemia, hyperbilirubinemia, and kernicterus in infants. Menadione should *not* be used to address vitamin K deficiency.[46] Also, don't take products containing vitamin K if you are taking anticoagulants (such as coumadin or warfarin) because vitamin K interferes with these drugs.

Vitamins C, A, and E were covered in chapter 6.

SOURCES FOR LIVE VITAMINS AND ORGANIC MINERALS

The challenge is to get healthy quantities of these vitamins and minerals. Although food sources are always best, if you think you can get enough vitamins and minerals to correct an imbalance by eating regular food in today's world, you might be sadly mistaken. For example, Michael Dobbins, D.C., reports, "Some researchers have said that as much as 90 percent of the calcium in pasteurized milk is not processed by the body."[47] Studies have linked the use of milk products "to a greater risk of coronary heart disease, other cardiovascular disease, cancer, diabetes, ulcerative colitis, lupus erythematosus, hypochromic microcytic anemia, kidney/bladder stones, female infertility, cataracts, gastrointestinal distress, colic, nasopharyngeal allergic reactions, and muscle cramps during pregnancy. Consumers also must consider the possibility of contamination from agricultural chemicals, synthetic hormones or disease-causing organisms in some dairy products," according to Bob LeRoy, R.D.[48]

Also, the soils in which foods are grown today are tremendously depleted of their vitamin and mineral content. In addition, many foods contain large amounts of pesticides or herbicides that can be toxic to bones (see chapter 11). Many foods also suffer from being overprocessed, which removes their remaining nutrients or renders them inert or unavailable.

These concerns have led to the idea of taking over-the-counter mineral supplements. However, they are not problem free either. One difficulty is that most are synthetic chemicals isolated from their cofactors, and therefore likely not to be assimilated. Another complication is deciding which chemical form to use; for example, calcium carbonate, or citrate, or what? Calcium carbonate is the synthetic form of calcium most widely purchased by consumers, but over-the-counter products are often difficult to absorb due to improper formulation. This form of calcium produces the white filmy ring that appears after boiling hard water. Synthetic limestone (when put into products, called dolomite) is generally insoluble. That means it requires stomach hydrochloric acid to break it down, and thus uses this acid up quickly. Dolomite has to undergo eleven biochemical changes to be absorbed, whereas the calcium lactate I took to heal my bones requires only two.[49]

Suppose you were walking along one day and picked up a stone from the ground. You took it to a laboratory to see what it was composed of, and the report came back saying it had 1,500 milligrams of calcium. If you then swallowed the stone, thinking you'd get your calcium dose for the day, you'd be sadly mistaken, for your body doesn't have a gizzard or some grinding machine to break down the stone and render the calcium available. Besides, if the calcium in the stone isn't accompanied by its helpers, your body won't be able to use much of it even if you could grind it down.

Many of the calcium products on the market are like that. A University of Maryland School of Pharmacy study in 1987 showed "that more than half of the eighty brands of calcium tablets tested . . . failed to meet the dissolution criteria."[50] This study was followed up by Consumers Union, which tested seven brands and found that four of the seven failed to meet USP (the U.S. Pharmacopoeia) standards. In many cases, the pills were coated with shellac, rendering them insoluble by stomach acid: "The resulting product tended to act much like a slick pebble."[51]

Consumer Reports states that researchers do not recommend dolomite or bone meal, either, because "in the past, some samples have been contaminated with lead." Lead interferes with the hormone progesterone, which regulates the rate at which new bone is built. Oyster shells are high in calcium content, but our bodies are unable to access it. Chelated calcium is also ineffective. *Consumer Reports* points out that "chelation purportedly improves absorption, but it actually does little more than raise the price."[52] They add that even if calcium supplements do meet USP standards, "You're better off getting your calcium from food."

Recently, products containing microcrystalline hydroxyapatite (MCHC) have become available. Extracts of whole bone, these products provide the trace minerals and protein matrix necessary for the proper use of calcium. However, because most are heat processed, the protein matrix is destroyed, rendering them fairly useless, nutritionally speaking. If you plan to use such a product, make sure it has been analyzed for lead content, a common contaminant of bone meal products. Standard Process products are cold processed, leaving the protein matrix in place, and are free of such contamination.

The form of calcium that the body can use most easily is calcium bicarbonate, which is given an electrical charge (ionized) through the action of enzyme systems. But calcium bicarbonate cannot be made into tablets, according to Standard Process's *Clinical Reference Guide*, "because as soon as you start drying the bicarbonate it changes to calcium carbonate."[53] The closest thing to it is calcium lactate. That's why so many practitioners stick to concentrated mineral and vitamin food products that are made from real foods and are bioactive and bioavailable. Then the body can readily, in one or two metabolic steps, deliver them to bone, where they are stored as dicalcium phosphate.[54]

Finally, before going on to nutritional protocols, a word about colloidal minerals. According to Dan Newell, C.N., "Colloidal means suspended. You could take rock and grind it and then suspend it within a fluid and it would be essentially the same as long as it did not pass through a semipermeable membrane when in solution. In sea kelp, the minerals are found in plants." Whatever their plant source, he adds, "The minerals have been organized and balanced by the plants themselves and were at one time in a colloidal state. Once they enter the body they are again in a colloidal state."[55] Therefore, the quality of a mineral product is not about whether or not the minerals in it are colloidal, i.e., suspended; it is about whether or not the minerals are bioactive, bioavailable, balanced, and unadulterated.

RESTORING MINERALS AND VITAMIN HELPERS

To restore your mineral and vitamin balance, your practitioner will create your protocol from products that combine nutrients to balance your body needs. The following whole food concentrates and herbal products provide minerals and vitamins for good bone health.

Protocols are made from a combination of products as determined by your health practitioner. In the product descriptions below, "SP" designates Standard Process formulations, and "MH" designates those made by MediHerb. The sources for herbal information are *Principles and Practice of Phytotherapy: Modern Herbal Medicine*, by Simon Mills and Kerry Bone, and *MediHerb Innovative Herbal Solutions Product Catalog 2001*, unless otherwise noted. All products mentioned but not described here are detailed in other chapters (see index).

Whole Food Concentrates

Bio-Dent (SP) is the protomorphogen extract (the DNA substrate) of bone used to rebuild bone, especially around the teeth. It supports bone repair following mechanical removal of infection. Donald Warren, D.D.S., reports that use of Bio-Dent tablets daily "results in a remineralization of incipient decays in approximately 50 percent of cases. At 10 per day, it has been shown to remineralize osteoporotic tempero-mandibular joints (TMJs) and the head of the femur."[56]

Biost (SP), one of two supplements Berle took, supports bones, teeth, and joints. It contains connective tissue protomorphogen and manganese. It supplies the phosphatase enzyme that the body uses to metabolize the raw materials that compose bony tissue.

Cal-Amo (SP) is used to acidify the body when it is alkaline, and therefore sluggish, including sluggish digestion. It is used when the body lacks chlorides (rather than lacking phosphates).

Calcifood (SP), the other supplement Berle took, contains in raw form the fiber and minerals for building bones and teeth, including calcium, phosphorus, protein, and trace minerals. It is formulated in part from cold-processed raw bone meal, which retains its biological enzymes. If the factors it contains are not being fully utilized, practitioners often add Biost.

Calcium Lactate (SP, vegetarian) is so named because it is made from lactic acid, not dairy. It contains calcium and magnesium in a five-to-one ratio and in a form that the body can digest and use easily. It is used to correct high phosphorus and low calcium imbalances, especially where dental caries and bone deterioration are occurring. It depresses high phosphorus levels. It helps improve all muscle functions, including those of the heart. It helps with fidgety, nervous energy, as in people who run high fevers. Calcium lactate may also be taken immediately at the onset of a cold, because infections easily take hold in a calcium-deficient environment. It can be taken independently of food, as it establishes its own pH in the stomach.[57]

If your phosphorus is too low and your calcium is too high, your body will be more alkaline. Alkalinity is involved in asthma, allergy, arthritis, bursitis, and infections as well as in mineral deposit formation. To acidify your body, practitioners may recommend products from grain food sources that leave an acid ash when metabolized. They act like the accelerator on a car and help the body speed up.

Calsol (SP, vegetarian) is a cereal source of calcium and phosphorus in a five-to-three ratio. It's a good source of phosphorus for vegetarians or lacto-vegetarians, and is a balanced product for their long-term use. It's also good for hyperirritability, hyperperistalsis, and muscular symptoms.[58]

Catalyn (SP) contains multiple vitamins, trace minerals, and living enzymes. It is the initial product that Dr. Royal Lee developed from substances that originate in the germ and seed portion of plants. Many practitioners feel that taking Catalyn and nothing else would eventually heal the body because it contains so many things that the body needs, some of which may still be unknown to science. Michael Dobbins, D.C., says, "You can't overdo Catalyn because it's perfectly balanced." He recommends it to keep children's immune systems healthy in place of immunizations.[59] (Also see chapter 9.) Dr. Dobbins adds that "people are so grossly underfed now that three Catalyn a day won't do it. They often require six to twelve a day and up." He recommends chewing it for best results.

Because it provides enzymes and trace minerals that may be absent from the soil (and therefore unavailable to the body), Catalyn can provide the missing ingredients that make a nutritional protocol work.

Chezyn (SP) contains trace minerals of organically chelated zinc, copper, and iron in a balanced ratio. The body sometimes needs all three minerals, which may become evident in symptoms such as acne, poor soft-tissue healing, blood-sugar disturbances, poor immune responses, and prostate disorders. Chezyn is also used to support the pancreas in people with pancreatitis.

Organic Minerals (SP) are used in conditions of acidosis to alkalinize the blood, and with people whose thyroid (T_4) pulse is too high (hyperthyroid). Organic Minerals are high in minerals, such as potassium and magnesium, that leave an alkaline ash. They function like the brakes on a car, helping to slow things down, as when the heart races and muscles twitch due to lack of potassium. The minerals support the parasympathetic nervous system, including the vagus nerve, which results in a calming effect. This product is made in part from alfalfa, which is one of the most deeply rooted plants and, therefore, contains minerals from the various strata of soil that the roots contact. Organic Minerals help the thyroid to rehydrate in situations where it has dehydrated, perhaps due to a viral infection.

Ostrophin PMG (SP) combines Calcium Lactate, Calcifood, and Cal-Ma Plus to support the parathyroid. According to Michael Dobbins, D.C., it "is lower in manganese and higher in raw bone meal, the little bit more that will often make the difference. It's a more complete package for bone or connective tissue repair, including osteoporosis."[60]

Phosfood (SP) may be recommended if you have a phosphorus deficiency and osteoarthritis, gall or kidney stones, or tartar on the teeth. It also helps to acidify the alkalinity of a high calcium state when the body lacks phosphates.

Phytolyn (SP) contains clinical concentrations of kale and brussels sprouts. It is an excellent source of calcium in addition to having powerful antioxidant properties. Its calcium is bonded to the plant-based enzymes necessary for easy absorption and assimilation. Its minerals are delivered to bone along with the green plant substances they require to bind them to the collagen net.

Source of Life (Nature's Plus, vegetarian) is a multiple vitamin product similar to Catalyn. It is called a whole food concentrate; however, it does contain some synthetic chemical isolates.

SP Complete (SP, vegetarian) is also a multiple vitamin product. It is made, not from synthetic chemicals, but from whole foods such as flax meal, whey protein, buckwheat juice, and kale. It offers a balance of essential macro- and micronutrients from plant sources. Together these nutrients support healthy cardiovascular, digestive, and nervous system function along with antioxidant protection for the cells. SP Complete is especially convenient for replacing vital nutrients often lost during the refining process of many of the foods we eat.

Herbal Products

Herbal solutions combine ingredients that support connective tissue together with those that provide the vitamins and minerals that bones need. Most of these herbs were covered in the previous chapter, while some are included in later chapters (boswellia, black cohosh, celery seed, ginger, nettle leaf, and turmeric). Two additional solutions that are specifically better in supporting connective tissue and bones are:

Fe-Max Iron Tonic (MH) is specifically formulated from a variety of herbs to provide easily absorbable vitamins and minerals. It supports the production of healthy blood, encourages healthy digestion, stimulates healthy circulation, and promotes overall vitality. It contains naturally occurring iron, folic acid, vitamins, and minerals.

Green Oats contain calcium, silicon, iron, and copper.

Providing magical minerals and their vitamin helpers is only part of the equation in the quest for perfect bones. Once absorbed, minerals and vitamins must be carried to the bone bank, a process covered in chapter 8.

EIGHT

Providing Courier Service:
Dry Bones and Essential Fatty Acids

HOW ASTONISHING that an adorable, twelve-pound miniature dachshund named Lulu could teach truly powerful lessons about the significance of the food group known as oils, or essential fatty acids (EFAs). Yet that was exactly what happened.

Lulu was living with a couple dozen other dogs like her. The breeder explained that Lulu, age four, was going to deliver a litter of puppies in a couple of weeks, and six weeks later, when they were weaned, we could have her. As it turned out, we didn't have to wait that long because Lulu gave birth prematurely. Of the two puppies, one was born dead. The other had such a severe cleft palate that it could not even be dropper fed, and it, too, soon succumbed. It turned out that Lulu had a history of not being able to sustain a pregnancy. The breeder was frustrated with the vet bill and no results, and was ready to let her go to another home.

But that was not the only clue that something was wrong. Picking her up to bring her home, I remarked that her coat was not shiny. The breeder responded by spraying something on Lulu's hair to make it appear lustrous. As we got in the car to leave, the breeder mentioned that an X-ray had shown that Lulu had a bony spur in her spine, small and asymptomatic at the moment, but likely to become a problem later.

Lulu seemed to adjust to her new life, but she showed no energy and no enthusiasm for anything—not a new bed, not food, not toys, not treats, and not games. Although my family spent considerable effort trying to get Lulu to wag her tail, she would not. In fact, she seemed to have no personality. I assumed that she was grieving for her puppies and let it go. She would become aroused and alarmed and bark from time to time, but she was never interested or curious. If I saw that behavior in a human, I would have said the person was clinically depressed. We poured on more love, gave her good food, and went on with life, until several months later, when she began an alarming pattern.

Standing in the middle of the room, not moving or being touched, she would scream as if in excruciating pain. The vet gave her an ugly prognosis: Lulu had severe back problems that went with the breed. Luckily there was another vet nearby who specialized in back surgery. He would place rods in her back, and she'd be able to move around with a roller-skate-like contraption that would support her from midbody down, while she pulled herself with her front legs. Now she wasn't the only one who felt depressed.

On impulse, as I was leaving for an appointment with a health care practitioner who does nutritional work, I took Lulu along. This practitioner's verdict was more hopeful. Lulu lacked certain oils. Add a teaspoon of olive oil a day to her diet, and she'd slowly get better. The bony spur would gradually be withdrawn back into the spinal vertebrae. Give it three months.

And that's exactly what happened. Every day Lulu became a little more mobile, a little more interested in life, more playful. By the third month, she ran and jumped and wagged her tail. Her natural, affectionate, happy personality came into full flower. She'd run to the kitchen where her treats were stored, wag her tail ferociously, point her nose at the treat box, and run back to the living room to arouse anyone who would listen. She even learned to roll over. She trotted happily along on six-mile hikes. She was back in the game of life, and she was playing to the fullest. And she stayed vigorous and full of zest until she finally died—of old age.

THE LIPID FOOD GROUP

Oils are such a significant part of the diet that the lack of them can produce such profound symptoms, while their addition can effect a truly powerful turnaround. Lulu's disintegration and recovery demonstrated some of the roles that essential fatty acids play in health disturbances: hormonal insufficiencies, lackluster or unhealthy skin and hair, energy production disturbances, depression, and calcium absorption and delivery problems sufficient to create bony spurs, back problems, and birth defects such as cleft palate.

I was to witness a human version of this in my practice when a therapist referred a woman of menopausal age whose major symptom was clinical depression but who did not want to take prescription antidepressants. Testing revealed that she was severely deficient in certain essential fatty acids. (It is likely that the demand for EFAs, which are the precursors to hormones, is higher during the menopausal shift.) Unfortunately, menopause is a time when many women are trying to force themselves to avoid fats in the interest of keeping their weight down and reducing heart disease risk. But heart disease is actually one outcome of a *lack* of EFAs.

Whatever the reason, this particular woman was so depleted in EFAs that she had to take triple the usual amount of four products containing a variety of EFAs: Black Currant Seed Oil, Chlorophyll Complex, Linum B_6, and Wheat Germ Oil (see below for descriptions). She pulled out of her depression in just a few days and stayed out of it by maintaining her intake of these essential fatty acids.

How could oils pull someone out of a depression? For one thing, essential fatty acids are precursors for hormones. Essential fatty acids are the building blocks of hormones in the same way that amino acids comprise proteins. EFAs may also reverse depression by providing fuel for the brain. According to Michael Dobbins, D.C., "The most efficient fuel for the brain is ketoacids, the breakdown products of fats."[1]

What are these powerful substances?

ESSENTIAL FATTY ACIDS

Fats or oils are also called "lipids," from the Greek word "lipos," which means fatlike substances. Membership in the lipid family is conferred on any nutrient that has the characteristic of being insoluble in water. It is a family whose relatives have some strange names. Some are called "true fats," which are esters of fatty acids and glycerol. Some are labeled "lipoids," such as phospholipids, cerebrosides, and waxes. Others are designated "sterols," such as cholesterol and ergosterol. Yet others are referred to as "hydrocarbons" and include squalene and carotene.[2]

Some members of this family of essential fatty acids, also called vitamin F, make excellent dinner guests, while their cousins, the saturated fats, have received a questionable reputation in the scientific community. And one branch of the family, transfatty acids, is clearly toxic and dangerous and best left uninvited.

The fatty acids to include are the polyunsaturated lipids that the body cannot make, but which it requires for every living cell. The parents of this healthy family are linoleic acid (omega-6) and linolenic acid (omega-3). They help maintain normal growth; their absence results in a lack of growth, as Lulu's puppies so painfully demonstrated. They also contribute to hormone production (including those hormones that sustain pregnancy to full term), proper digestion, and wound healing. Their presence improves the health of skin and hair. In fact, it is likely that there would be far less incidence (thirty-two thousand cases in 1997[3]) of malignant melanoma (skin cancer) if people were not so deficient in vitamin F, the essential fatty acids. According to James Balch, M.D., and Phyllis Balch, C.N.C., EFAs also "reduce blood pressure, aid in the prevention of arthritis, lower cholesterol and triglyceride levels, and reduce the risk of blood clot formation."[4]

But that's not all. EFAs are also central to optimal brain and nerve function. Balch and Balch point out that "a deficiency of essential fatty acids can lead to an impaired ability to learn and recall information."[5] In part, that's because key brain nutrients must be carried to the brain in oil form in order to pass the protective blood-brain barrier. Also, the neurotransmitters the brain requires are made of EFAs. And, the layer of insulation around the nerves, the myelin sheath, is composed of fats (such as cholesterol, cerebrosides, phospholipids, and certain fatty acids).[6] Without this protection, nerves cannot carry impulses from one place to another; instead, they misfire in a disorganized fashion.

This is a danger of cholesterol levels that are too low. Indeed, lower cholesterol levels are "associated with a greater risk of death from cancer and respiratory and digestive diseases," according to Kerri Bodmer and Nan Fuchs.[7] Perhaps that is why the existence of some brain seizure disturbances has been linked either to a deficiency of EFAs or a disturbance in their metabolism. Children with hyperactivity and attention problems have, according to Hunter Yost, M.D., "been found to be deficient in omega-3 relative to omega-6 fatty acids." Likewise, excessive anxiety and mood instability in adults may result from an imbalance between "good" and "bad" prostaglandins, a disequilibrium due in part to overconsumption of hydrogenated oils.[8]

EFAs—the welcome dinner guests (sometimes also called "cis form")—are made up of two groups: omega-3, or alpha-linolenic acid, and omega-6, including linoleic and gamma-linoleic acid. Omega-3

EFAs are found in vegetable oils such as flax and chia seeds, walnut, pumpkin seed, canola oil, and fish oil. Omega-6 EFAs are found in unsaturated vegetable oils such as soybean, primrose, sesame, grape seed, and borage. They are also contained in legumes, raw nuts, and seeds.

Most food sources contain a mix of both types of essential fatty acids. But the one plant with the highest amount of EFAs, rich in omega-3 and omega-6, is hemp. Hemp is a cousin of the cannabis plant, but unlike marijuana it contains no THC. It is more like hop or nettle, two other members of its family.[9] A source of these desirable EFAs that is relatively new to Americans is emu oil, either from California or imported from Australia.

Whatever their source, EFAs support the body's defenses against high cholesterol, high blood pressure, rheumatoid arthritis, and heart disease as well as helping decrease allergic responses and dissolve tumors. Omega-6s contain lignans, which intestinal bacteria change into compounds that are highly protective against cancer, especially breast cancer. Additionally, lignans are antibacterial, antifungal, and antiviral.

Michael Dobbins, D.C., points out that omega-6 fatty acids, such as those found in red meats, organ meats, and dairy fats, increase swelling (they produce arachidonic acid). However, when people consume no omega-6s, such as strict vegetarians, their liver gets a signal that more is needed and makes more. The result can be increased cholesterol levels.[10]

To address high cholesterol problems, some companies are now manufacturing epoprostenol, or prostacyclin, which is synthetically produced to attempt to reverse vascular lesions. But a better answer, emphasizes Dr. Dobbins, is to balance the ecosanoid system, which metabolizes essential fatty acids, by proper eating. What might that mean?

Mary Jane Mack, R.N., recommends olive oil, canola oil, and butter. She emphasizes that people on low-fat or no-fat diets have the most health problems. "There's no lubrication in their bodies. They are open for osteoporosis because they lack the nutrients the body needs to function at a healthy state. Fat is necessary."[11] Dr. Dobbins concurs. "The higher the fat intake, the lower the incidence of breast cancer, according to the nurses' study, which included eighteen thousand cases."[12]

Lipids contribute to health first by supplying a continuous source of fuel that the body can use or store through a process called thermogenesis, which increases oxygen taken in by cells. Any time that extra energy is needed, the body can call on stores of these oils for energy. That's why competitive athletes add EFAs to their diet, and Alaskan sled-dog mushers add flax seed oil, rich in EFAs, to their dogs' diets. These oils spare protein cell walls and cell nuclei from being broken down for energy production. Additionally, essential fatty acids help the body absorb all the fat-soluble vitamins: A, D, E, and K.

The right balance of EFAs, says Ann Louise Gittleman, M.S., "will allow you to lose weight effortlessly and painlessly without becoming preoccupied with dieting. . . . Essential fat is the healthiest and easiest way to attain and maintain your normal weight."[13]

Essential fatty acids and bone health go hand in glove. EFAs can be thought of as the armored trucks that carry payloads of minerals to their destination, the bone bank. According to the *Clinical Reference Guide*, "Vitamin F [these essential fatty acids] maintains a gut calcium level for the vitamin D to draw upon. Vitamin D can then pull the calcium out of the stomach and into the blood, and the vitamin F carries it from the blood to the tissues and bones."[14]

But EFAs can't do their job in certain circumstances, such as when too many saturated fats are present. The reputation of saturated fats has suffered a great deal lately, for rumor had it that they were a chief cause of coronary artery disease. This idea is becoming increasingly unlikely as evidence to the contrary is amassed. For example, the Eskimo diet that was studied was 80 percent fat for most of the year, and most of that fat saturated.[15] How could they have survived so long if saturated fats were so bad?

Still, the body does have to use up unsaturated fats to process saturated ones, so at the very least, saturated fats need to be balanced with sufficient unsaturated ones. Otherwise the oils that should be carrying calcium to bones are so busy getting rid of saturated fats that they never get down to the task of transporting new calcium stores to harden bones. An additional problem is that, due to modern farming methods, saturated fats can contain pesticide residues that interfere "with nerve function and oxidation processes in the human body," according to Mary Frost, M.A.[16]

The outcasts of the family of oils, because they are toxic, are called transfatty acids. They result when hydrogen is forced into polyunsaturated oil molecules using high temperature and pressure, or when vegetable oils are constantly reused, as with deep-fried foods at fast food restaurants. Transfatty acids are found in margarine and any other product labeled "partially hydrogenated" or "hydrogenated."

Evidence is mounting that links these transfatty acids to a variety of health problems, including heart disease and cancer. The mass commercial refinement of oils has stripped EFAs from the diet and interfered with the formation of certain essential fatty acids that prevent tissue destruction and promote healing (in particular, prostaglandins).[17] Michael Dobbins, D.C., points out that "transfats block the cascade of metabolic breakdown. They confuse the body; it uses the transfat instead of the good fat."[18]

Some supplements, such as borage oil, evening primrose oil, and black currant seed oil, can bypass the transfat intake problem. However, EFA production can still be stopped by isolated fragments of nutrients like vitamin E or aspirin.[19]

The body uses essential fatty acids to make a variety of necessary substances. One of these is a steroid called cholesterol, which has recently suffered a bad reputation also. But it is truly a required component of cell membranes, where it helps regulate the transfer of nutrients and waste products. Cholesterol is naturally produced by the liver in a process that insulin levels control. It is therefore the rise and fall of insulin levels associated with refined carbohydrates that seems to deserve the bad reputation currently pinned on saturated fats. Once manufactured, cholesterol is used as a fundamental building block for hormones and a coating for nerve fibers.

The body also uses EFAs to make over two hundred kinds of prostaglandins, most of which are manufactured in the liver. They are hormone-like substances that serve as chemical messengers to help regulate the functions of cells. Prostaglandins control a variety of bodily processes, including arterial muscle tone, sodium excretion, blood platelet inflammatory responses, and various immune functions.[20] Each process needs to work in concert with the others. If one is out of balance, it can shut down the entire system.[21]

Certain fats promote inflammation. These inflammation-promoting fats exist in red meats, liver, dairy fats, shellfish, and certain vegetable oils such as peanut, safflower, and corn oils. Other fats are inflammation inhibiting; these are found in foods such as olive oil, canola oil, evening primrose oil, borage, black currant seed oil, gooseberries, spirulina, flaxseed, English walnut, soybeans, wheat germ, chestnuts, spinach, and beans. This second type of fat is helpful in reducing inflammatory conditions, including arthritis.

The role of essential fatty acids in producing healthy bones cannot be overestimated. It's completely straightforward: no essential fatty acids, no healthy bones. EFAs carry the minerals and their vitamin helpers that bones need. And EFAs are necessary ingredients to produce every hormone that directs bone bank activities. It is little wonder, then, that the incidence of osteoporosis is linked with insufficient dietary intake of essential fatty acids.

Porous bones are among the dangers of a low-fat diet, especially when the small amount of fat eaten is saturated. A low-fat diet exposes the body to the danger of having no carriers to convey new mineral deposits into the bone bank. Of course, there are numerous other associated problems, such as liver trouble and immune system breakdown. For women, insufficient body fat mass is dangerous to bones. When body fat mass is reduced to around 15 percent, the menses may stop and bone loss (from low fat mass) begins. But insufficient fat content in the diet can also damage the immune system, a fact that Nathan Pritikin, M.D., found out. He lowered his body fat to 2 or 3 percent and his dietary fat intake to nearly zero in an attempt to avoid heart disease, only to die of leukemia. One wonders how his immune system could function with no essential fatty acids.

But too much intake of dietary fat can also be problematic. It appears that high fat intake, when associated with highly refined carbohydrates, contributes to a high incidence of heart disease. In terms of bone health, too much fat intake creates a high level of acids in the bodily fluids. To neutralize these acids, the body draws calcium out of bones. Thus, long-term high-fat intake equals a greater likelihood of osteoporosis.

One attempt to deal with this problem has resulted in the manufacture of fake fats. One is called Olean, with the trademark name of Olestra. According to the Center for Science in the Public Interest, (CSPI), Olean has been shown to cause diarrhea, loose stools, intestinal cramping, and other gastrointestinal symptoms including fecal incontinence. Some people have even been hospitalized as a result of these symptoms. Additionally, fake fats rob the body of nutrients, in part by interfering with the absorption of carotenoids, a family of fat-soluble nutrients that have been associated with lowering the risk of cardiovascular disease and cancer. Nonetheless, the Food and Drug Administration has approved the use of Olean.[22]

Some fatty metabolism problems are due, not to insufficient or excessive intake, but rather to interference with their complete break-down. Such disruption can occur in bulimia as a result of a pH shift. Interference with the complete breakdown of EFAs can also occur from taking anti-inflammatory substances such as aspirin, nonsteroidal anti-inflammatory drugs (NSAIDS), epolipoic acid (EPA), and high doses of *synthetic* (but not whole food) vitamin E. They all inhibit the breakdown of oils into their final metabolic products (specifically the PG 1, 2, and 3 prostaglandin series). Because these substances are incompletely metabolized, they contribute to the inflammatory process, requiring more and more dependence on the anti-inflammatory substances that prevented their complete metabolism in the first place. And the body is deprived of the metabolic materials that would have been available and that it needs for other maintenance and rebuilding projects.

Still other fatty metabolism problems are associated with environmental circumstances that place a high demand for them, for example, drying environments such as those near chemical plants, nuclear power plants, or exposure to extreme weather. Apparently these oils are burned up rapidly in such surroundings. People show the same initial symptoms as with an EFA deficiency. People become creaky and stiff and freeze up, like the Tin Woodsman in *The Wizard of Oz*. They also build up sludge in the blood. In the human body, as in motor vehicles, oils lubricate all the parts, help keep them moving, and keep the body clean by carrying away refuse. Lack of EFAs is also a common finding in men with prostate cancer, for which practitioners often recommend Linum B_6 (see below).

Unfortunately, essential fatty acids are extremely volatile. According to Michael Dobbins, D.C., "In their naturally occurring form, fats kink into a spiral, which means a great deal of exposure to the air; thus, they have a high oxygenation rate and can easily become rancid."[23] When exposed to heat or air, these spiral-shaped fats partially decompose, in the process forming free radicals that are dangerous to cellular health.

Nutritionist Royal Lee, D.D.S., pointed out one example. He said that lecithin is a source of essential fatty acids. It contains essential fatty acids called phospholipids, which are hormone precursors that enable our glandular system to function. However, he emphasized, if lecithin is refined, it actually promotes bone decalcification.[24]

Therefore, how the food industry processes these oils has everything to do with their actual nutritional content once ingested. Unfortunately, most commercially prepared oils today are subject to a type of processing that negatively affects their nutrient value. Mary Frost, M.A., states, "Expeller-pressed oils and hydraulic-pressed oils are first subjected to temperatures of 200 degrees F and up. The oils are then de-gummed, which removes chlorophyll, vitamin E, lecithin, and many minerals and trace elements. Then an alkaline wash separates out even more nutrients. Next, the oil is bleached and then deodorized by steam distillation at temperatures over 450 degrees F."[25] This oil then can be labeled "cold pressed," a term that has no legal meaning.

However, the body knows the difference. No matter what amount of processed oils are consumed, the bottom line is that the body begins to break down because it simply does not have the essential fatty acids it needs to carry out crucial functions.

Given how central essential fatty acids are to health, low levels of EFAs in the population should be considered a public health problem. According to Hunter Yost, M.D., "Breast milk and infant formula in this country have been found to have lower levels of the essential fatty acids omega-3 . . . as compared to European breast milk and formula. This fatty acid is necessary for proper brain and eye development in infants and mood regulation in adults."[26] And Donald Rudin, M.D., reports that his research conclusion is that "Americans consume only 20% of the EFAs required for optimal health. Thus we crave food rich in fat and eat the wrong kind."[27]

Indeed, EFA levels have been demonstrated to be significantly lower in people with heart disease than in those who are healthy.[28]

Does the significance of essential fatty acids to bone health mean we should immediately increase our intake? No, not quite so fast. There is one essential prerequisite: the body has to be able to absorb and process them, which involves the gallbladder.

PROCESSING ESSENTIAL FATTY ACIDS

The gallbladder is a small sac located just under the right rib cage. One of the gallbladder's functions is to concentrate the bile manufactured by the liver and release it in sufficient quantities at the proper digestive moment. It must function optimally for fats to be properly digested. If the gallbladder is performing poorly or if the liver's bile production is faulty, oils will not be properly metabolized. Then the oils cannot do two of their essential jobs: carry calcium to bones and rid the body of old minerals, metals, and toxins.

The gallbladder's stores help break down and emulsify fat from food and also help eliminate toxins. John Courtney from Standard Process provides an example: "If you create a lot of dust or if you work in a flour mill and breathe flour, it goes into your lungs where your blood picks it up and carries it over to the liver. The liver is like the oil filter in a car. It removes toxins from the blood and dumps them out of the body through the bile . . . which takes them to the intestines for elimination."[29]

This process has been demonstrated by following the path of injected radioactive charcoal into the bloodstream with a Geiger counter. Courtney adds, "If the bile gets thick like cream and does not flow smoothly, this indicates the person's fat metabolism is deficient. This is a symptom of gallbladder trouble. So we must thin the bile."[30]

The gallbladder's job is to retrieve all the minerals from the liver — including calcium, metals, and toxins—and then get rid of them. If it doesn't, it makes stones out of the minerals that it couldn't eliminate.

Improving gallbladder health was the first layer of healing for me to restore my bone health. It was also the first big problem that Carol Gieg began to correct after I first saw her. Had we begun increasing our intake of essential fatty acids before correcting our gallbladder functioning, we might have become sick indeed. Carol used Betafood (SP; see below) to help her condition.

That this protocol is effective can be seen in the reaction she had. A day or two after she began the protocol, Carol reported an intensified muscle soreness. This was likely a result of her body now playing catch-up: finishing the job of metabolizing what it could not complete before. That is why a low dose had been recommended for a week, so she wouldn't throw her body into a massive toxic reaction.

Actually, her response was good news, a sign that her bodily processes were getting back to work. Without this oil-metabolizing process working well, she would not be able to heal her bones.

Gallbladder functioning was also a problem for Sophia Tampinelli. As you may recall, her gallbladder had been surgically removed six years prior to her interview for this book. She'd had a big stone that had bothered her for years. However, after the surgery, she gained over sixty pounds, her bone health continued to deteriorate, and the underlying problem of bile formation remained unresolved. Since there was no gallbladder to retrieve waste metals and store bile, her liver tried to do so. After her liver could no longer do the job, she suffered increased symptoms of indigestion: bloating, gas, belching, her abdomen holding water, food allergies, emphysema, psoriasis, and even Crohn's disease (an intestinal inflammation). These symptoms were all a result of waste backup up in her liver.

A real house of cards can come tumbling down when the liver is backed up. It starts when unmetabolized oils turn to cholesterol, which is one of the primary reasons people have high cholesterol. The liver's job is so tremendously important that any conceivable disease, including osteoporosis, can be brought on when it shuts down. For example, the liver is a backup storehouse from which bone marrow can draw essential vitamins and minerals. The spleen backs up the liver. If the spleen, too, gets overwhelmed and shuts down, the body not only robs the bone marrow, it also has to work harder to repair the blood cells that the spleen's not repairing. The better the spleen works, the better the bone marrow.

Crystal M. had the unfortunate distinction of finding out the truth about the gallbladder's connection to bone health: "My gallbladder has probably not been working optimally all my life," she said. "I have been plagued with constipation since birth. As a young woman in my late twenties, digestive and other problems prompted a chiropractor to recommend a gallbladder cleanse. The regimen involved fasting, taking powerful laxatives, and ingesting a mixture of olive oil and citrus juice. It worked. I eliminated more than a cup of stones as large as marbles. It was painful, but not horrible. I tried it again several other times but had to stop."

However, Crystal's problem was still not solved. She continued to have light stools, a classic sign of gallbladder problems. She continues, "Along the way I learned to reduce or eliminate fatty foods due to the pain and problems they caused [which no doubt contributed significantly to her lack of essential fatty acids]. In the meantime, by age forty-five I developed severe osteoporosis. My nutritional consultant explained to me that essential fatty acids are needed to carry calcium to the bones. Lo and behold, during a nutritional evaluation, my gallbladder emerged as needing support. [For this she took Betafood (see below). She also needed Choline (see chapter 11) for support for the gallstones.] Luckily, with this protocol I never had a crisis. It took longer than I'd expected, but it worked. Now I am able to ingest important oils and move on to the next level of healing."

Now that Crystal's body has these EFAs, it can begin to repair her hormonal system. The hormonal system, which is Crystal's next layer of healing, is addressed in the next chapter.

So how can these essential fatty acids, the precursors to hormones, be provided, and how can their assimilation be assured?

Michael Dobbins, D.C., describes one way that health professionals can test for an imbalance in essential fatty acids. After placing a tablet of pure aspirin (acetylsalicylic acid) under someone's tongue, they test an indicator muscle that has been weak. If the muscle strengthens, it indicates a severe ecosanoid system (EFA) imbalance. The test works because the acetyl group in aspirin cuts the production of the entire ecosanoid system, including those aspects that are involved in pain perception.

Dr. Dobbins adds that when the body indicates such an imbalance, practitioners recommend dietary changes. For example, restricting carbohydrates, as recommended in *Dr. Atkins' New Diet Revolution,* is the fastest way to rebalance the ecosanoid system. Restricting carbohydrates quickly balances brain chemistry, which allows neurotransmitters to get going again.

Dr. Dobbins emphasizes that fatty acids are the optimum food, "the big log on the fire that keeps you warm all night," whereas carbohydrates are "like kindling."[31] When carbohydrates and fats are consumed at the same time, the body deals first with the one more readily oxidized, the carbohydrate, and stores the fat from calories we don't need in triglyceride form. "If you then eat more carbohydrates, the body doesn't get back to burning the triglyceride it stored. So the problem was never fat; it was not getting back to the fat to burn it." The solution, he says, is to get on a high-fat, high-protein ketogenic (fat-burning) diet. He reports that "one woman came into his office with triglycerides at 1,400, immediately went on such a diet, and her levels fell to 200 in forty-eight hours."[32] Practitioners may also recommend supplementation with black currant seed oil and wheat germ oil.

However, when the liver has been shut down for a long time, reactivating it to carry out its role in EFA metabolism can be difficult. For this problem, Super-Eff (see below) is often recommended. It provides EFAs that don't require the liver to break them down. When the liver recovers, it will again be able to process EFAs on its own.

RESTORING ESSENTIAL FATTY ACIDS

Resupplying the body with essential fatty acids can improve bone health dramatically, and in the process, may also improve conditions such as eczema, PMS, sterility, poor wound healing, arthritis, mood swings, seizure disorders, hormone imbalance, and cancer. The following products supply EFAs.

Protocols are made from a combination of products as determined by your health practitioner. In the product descriptions below, "SP" designates Standard Process formulations, and "MH" designates those made by MediHerb. The sources for herbal information are *Principles and Practice of Phytotherapy: Modern Herbal Medicine*, by Simon Mills and Kerry Bone, and *MediHerb Innovative Herbal Solutions*

Product Catalog 2001, unless otherwise noted. All products mentioned but not described here are detailed in other chapters (see index).

Whole Food Concentrates

A-F Betafood (SP) contains Betafood (see below) with Cataplex A and Cataplex F, which provide additional support for detoxification.

Betafood (SP, vegetarian) provides nutritional support to aid in the digestion and absorption of essential fatty acids. It is designed to flush the entire route through which bile flows and thus eliminate toxins brought to the liver to be filtered out. If bile gets too thick, it can't flow easily, which indicates that fat metabolism is deficient. Betafood contains concentrated beet juice to help decongest the liver, mobilize bile, and provide methyl donors, which can create additional chemical-compound bonding sites and thus aid fat metabolism. Taking six Betafood a day has the cleansing power of eating twenty beets a day.

Black Currant Seed Oil (SP) is concentrated from cold-processed black currant seeds. It has a high quantity of gamma linolenic acid (GLA), a converted form of linolenic acid produced in the liver if it is healthy. It is superior to evening primrose oil as a source of GLAs. GLA is used up rapidly in people who have inflammatory processes for any reason, whether from working out a lot, from arthritis, or from food sensitivity. GLA is also needed when someone has eczema or very dry skin, for "the body is not converting essential fatty acids into the form that the sebaceous glands under the skin use, which is GLA."[33] Evening primrose oil contains these oils, but in a lesser concentration, making it less potent to rapidly improve bodily stores.

Cataplex F (SP) tablets are a source of essential polyunsaturated fatty acids, primary arachidonic acid. The EFAs they contain also include some of arachidonic acid's parents, linoleic and linolenic acid. They help transport calcium from blood to tissues. The EFAs ionize calcium lactate to make it available to the tissues. Cataplex F also contains some protein-bound iodine, and therefore also supports the thyroid, hair, skin, and nails. It is used for calcium starvation, calcium assimilation problems, herpes simplex, hypothyroidism, ridged nails, poor hair quality, dry skin, muscle cramps, hypervitaminosis D, sunburn, sun poisoning, sun sensitivity, heat prostration, and prostate problems.

The EFAs in Cataplex F provide the balance to vitamin D, as described previously. The EFAs help spread calcium into the tissues, especially in any condition when the body's surface (i.e., skin or nails) has become hard or brittle.[34] Standard Process F Perles (gelatin capsules) are excellent for dry bones. They are vitamin F in the oil form (Linum B_6), essential fatty acids. Cataplex F Perles (SP) are similar to Cataplex F tablets, but they contain no iodine.

Chlorophyll Complex (SP) is a fat-soluble chlorophyll and therefore retains fat-soluble nutrients, especially vitamins A, E, F, and K. Chlorophyll Complex is a also a source of vitamin K, which helps produce fibrin, important in the clotting mechanism. The structure of the chlorophyll molecule is very close to that of hemoglobin, which carries oxygen to the tissues. The main difference is that magnesium is primary in chlorophyll molecules, where iron is present in hemoglobin. Therefore this product is often used for anemia as well as being a source of EFAs and of the fat-soluble vitamins A, D, E, and K.

Bruce West, D.C., states, "It's a rare instance when I do not recommend a Chlorophyll Complex Perle for anyone suffering from kidney stones or osteoporosis. Chlorophyll activates a blood protein called osteocalcin, which is critical for the proper formation of bone. Without this activity you cannot build bone [which can lead to osteoporosis] and you develop the chronic formation of calcium oxalate (the major form of kidney stones)." He instructs people to think of this chlorophyll product "when you need to move calcium and other minerals into your bones and out of your kidneys. Chlorophyll is the substance that absorbs trace minerals like boron and molybdenum from soil and gets them into plants. When you consume chlorophyll, you are getting a host of trace minerals and a supreme source of organic magnesium . . . the natural balance for calcium, especially when it comes to kidney stones."[35]

Dr. West insists on using a chlorophyll product that is truly cold processed, not merely labeled so, which is why he recommends Standard Process. His reasoning is that "there are enzymes in and around the fat soluble chlorophyll molecule that the body needs to build bones from all the other materials which heat processing destroys. If lacking the enzymes, which most people are, they won't build bone properly. Also, few people get a good source of raw fat."[36]

Evening Primrose Oil (MH) contains essential fatty acids from the omega-6 series, which make it excellent for reducing prostaglandin-induced inflammation by providing gamma linolenic acid (GLA), a precursor for prostaglandin E_1. Some sources suggest that its GLAs are more bioavailable than other GLA-containing sources. Experiments with rats have demonstrated that those fed a diet high in GLAs and EPAs (in a ratio of three to one) had significantly increased bone calcium content.[37, 38]

Linum B$_6$ (SP) is "organically grown fresh flaxseed oil. . . . Cold processed [in the right way that preserves their structure and not just labeled so] . . . especially high in linolenic acid . . . the most fragile of all oils . . . it goes rancid so easily." It is high in omega-3 fatty acids, which are typically deficient in the American diet. "Flaxseed oil is less likely to be polluted when organically grown than fish oils, which are also high in omega-3 fatty acids. An omega-3 deficiency is signified by sticky platelets."[39] Linum B$_6$ contains the vitamin F oils that are the natural antagonist to vitamin D.[40]

Sesame Seed Oil (SP) contains concentrated vitamin T, which stands for thrombocyte, a blood cell that aids in coagulating blood. This vitamin is often low in people who have a low thrombocyte count, such as in leukemia, and severe blood conditions, including anemia. In fact, one Midwestern doctor had three children who overcame leukemia by eating six tablespoonfuls of brown sesame butter (which contains high concentrations of the oil) a day.[41] Vitamin T feeds the bone marrow some of the raw building materials it needs to raise the red blood cell count.

Super-Eff (SP) is used to provide arachidonic acid when the liver cannot produce it from breaking down essential fatty acids. It provides EFA breakdown products directly for people whose condition is severely degenerated, as in muscular dystrophy or multiple sclerosis.

Wheat Germ Oil (SP) can eliminate muscle cramps that are due to the body's failure to deliver calcium to the muscles. It also contains sex hormone precursors, and is therefore good for hot flashes. This product also contains a vitamin recognized in England, but not in the United States, called "B$_4$." Vitamin B$_4$ has been known to correct arrhythmias of the heart.[42] Additionally, Wheat Germ Oil is excellent for keeping fallopian tubes and the vas deferens healthy, as it helps keep these tubes from collapsing. It's also used to help repair scar tissue. Some practitioners suggest rubbing it directly onto the scar tissue.

In acute situations involving gallstones, practitioners often recommend a combination of products every fifteen minutes, which may include: Choline (see chapter 11), Betafood, Linum B$_6$, and Phosfood (see chapter 7).[43]

Vegetarian protocols for the gallbladder generally include Betafood, sometimes with the addition of Choline, and Betaine Hydrochloride. Protocols for liver support are in chapter 11.

Herbal Products

Burdock (MH) is a liquid extract often used to support healthy liver and gallbladder function. It supports healthy blood, boosts the immune system and the body's natural resistance function, and helps keep skin healthy.

Dandelion Root (MH) is a liquid extract that helps support healthy liver and gallbladder function by supporting bile production to digest fats, and by assisting the liver in naturally filtering and neutralizing accumulated toxins. It also encourages natural function among the body's major organs of elimination. These benefits are derived from the root, not the leaves.

Globe Artichoke (MH) is a liquid extract that contains various phyto-chemicals that support healthy liver and gallbladder function and help maintain cholesterol levels within a normal range. The phyto-chemicals also promote a proper intestinal environment and stimulate digestion. In addition, they encourage healthy fluid levels and help maintain healthy blood.

Livton Complex (MH) tablets contain a blend of globe artichoke, dandelion root, milk thistle, fringe tree, and greater celandine, which together help support a healthy liver, gallbladder, digestive system, bowel, and organs of elimination and also help maintain healthy blood.

Turmeric (MH) is a liquid extract that contains an essential oil along with yellow pigments that support healthy liver function and bile secretion and support the proper breakdown of dietary fats. In addition, it provides antioxidant protection, promotes normal platelet function and circulation, promotes the body's normal protective response to environmental stresses, and maintains and supports healthy joints.

Once essential fatty acids are absorbed and metabolized, the body can begin to use their breakdown products to manufacture the substances that regulate the bone bank. These regulators are the powerful hormones, the subject of chapter 9.

NINE

Regulating the Bank: Hormones for Bones

WHEN HORMONE IMBALANCES are involved in osteoporosis, it carries the medical diagnosis of "Type I" osteoporosis. But hormones seem a world away from bones. What does one have to do with the other?

Hormones are the governing officers of the bone bank, regulating all its activity. The pituitary gland is the president of the board. It secretes hormones that oversee and direct the activities of all the board members, the other endocrine glands. These include adrenals, thyroid, parathyroid, pineal, pancreas, liver, male gonadal (prostate and testes) or female gonadal (ovaries, uterus, and mammary), duodenum, thymus, and the power behind the scenes, the hypothalamus. Together they set policies and give directives for the bone bank. Hormones hold the power to determine whether to increase, maintain, or withdraw deposits from bones. And hormones are potent substances; they achieve their objectives even in very small amounts.

The word "hormone" is derived from the Greek *hormon*, meaning to arouse or excite. Technically, hormones are chemical substances made in an organ or gland. Once manufactured, though, they are conveyed through the blood to another part of the body. It is at these target sites that they demonstrate their regulatory command, stimulating some activities and reducing others.

Some hormones are more important to the bone bank than others. For example, hormones made by the uterus, prostate, and parathyroid gland help the bone marrow produce and release various minerals. Three other hormones (parathyroid hormone, dihydroxy-vitamin D, and calcitonin from the thyroid gland) control blood calcium levels. Together these hormones supervise calcium: how much is absorbed by the intestine, excreted through the kidneys, and taken into bones. Still other hormones (parathormone and progesterone) regulate the deposit of calcium into tissues. To produce these hormones, the body requires essential fatty acids (EFAs). Therefore, an insufficient level of EFAs can create hormone imbalances and deregulate the bone bank.

Assuming enough raw materials to make sufficient hormones, each hormone factory or gland raises its voice on the governing board relative to its particular assignments. In turn, the release of each potent hormonal substance must be timed and integrated with all the others to produce perfect bones. For example, the ovaries or testicles produce hormones stored in the uterus or prostate, and the pituitary gland organizes them together and with parathyroid.

Hormone production problems are all related to each other; if one lags in production, other board members try to cover their buddy's job. For example, if ovaries or testes are removed or malfunctioning, adrenal glands strive to produce the missing sex hormones. Since the missing glands help metabolize calcium, the parathyroid tries to back up that function.

One hormone imbalance can affect other hormone factories like one domino falling in a line of dominoes. Dan Newell, C.N., describes what happens: "The pH normalizing glands are the adrenals and thyroid. When these prime regulators of pH balance are affected, they go into overdrive trying to regulate. When that's been going on for some time, and then the menopausal hormone shift is added to the hormone factories' work load, the pituitary enlarges. The pituitary tries to compensate for the lack of ovarian hormones. Most women notice a headache over their left ear."[1] First the adrenals fail because they're overstressed. The thyroid tries to back them up, but gets tired too. Then the pituitary overworks. By the time the hormonal shift of menopause takes place, the whole line of dominoes can start tumbling down.

THE HORMONAL SYSTEM

Each hormone on the board not only has particular allies, but also has antagonists that can oppose their activities. To better understand how health practitioners use clinical nutrition to support the hormonal system, a brief introduction to each hormone is given below. Each hormone has a unique contribution to running the bone bank, and therefore to the quest for perfect bones.

Pituitary

The pituitary gland is tiny, no bigger than a hickory nut but nonetheless wields tremendous power. It sits at the base of the brain, where it chairs the board of bone bank regulators. This leadership position is well-deserved, for the pituitary produces more hormones than any other gland: hormones that stimulate growth, sexual development, the reproductive cycle, digestion, metabolism, water intake and output, lactation, blood pressure, and even labor contractions. For these contributions, the pituitary has earned the title "the master gland."

Someone whose pituitary is chronically weak during childhood may grow to be short in stature. But a weak pituitary can also result in an overly acidic stomach. When the pituitary develops an acute weakness, as when it orchestrates the profound hormonal shifts of menopause, it can change metabolism, raise blood pressure, and create disturbances in water intake and output, contributing to hot flashes and night sweats.

The pituitary's allies on the governing board—other hormone factory members who will cooperate quickly and supportively when a job needs to be done—are the thyroid, gonads, mammary, and adrenal glands.

In case the pituitary gets out of hand, perhaps too power hungry or not knowing when to quit, two other board members will antagonize it: the pancreas and the duodenum. If necessary, these two junior board members can cause a complete insurrection.

Thyroid

The thyroid is a horseshoe-shaped gland residing at the front of the neck. It makes a variety of hormones. Bruce West, D.C., refers to it as the "middleman for the way your body balances calcium."[2]

The thyroid gland also makes T_3, which controls the rhythm of the kidneys. When insufficient T_3 is produced, the person may develop incontinent bowel because they have too many fluids in the body.

T_4, another hormone the thyroid produces, controls the rhythm of the heart; therefore, deficient levels can cause symptoms such as fatigue, depression, headaches, and cold extremities due to poor circulation. T_4 deficiency can also result in goiters, double chins, and symptoms that mimic heart failure.[3]

The relationship of thyroid hormones to bone health is a central one: thyroid hormones are required for bone remodeling to take place. "Thyroid hormone is one of the triggers for the bone-remodeling cycle, which starts with bone resorption and is followed by new bone formation. If not enough thyroid hormone is present, old bone tends to accumulate—bone that is not necessarily strong or fracture-resistant," says Alan Gaby, M.D.[4]

When the thyroid is out of balance, people can get crabby very quickly. Clinical nutritionist and researcher Dan Newell, C.N., estimates that he has helped several hundred menopausal women rebalance their endocrine systems by providing nutritional support for their thyroids. He says that some women undergoing menopause develop increased thyroid activity, which causes a faster withdrawal rate from the bone bank (a faster turnover in osteoclast activity). The parathyroid also kicks into high gear to get rid of the calcium that was drawn into the blood from the bones. These women exhibit muscular weakness over the scapula (the upper shoulder area) in the back. The focus of nutritional support is to calm down the thyroid (see the protocols below). Probably about 50 to 60 percent of patients respond to this kind of approach, he adds.[5]

The thyroid's major supporters are the adrenal glands, the pituitary gland, and the gonads (ovaries or testes). The liver is also central to thyroid functioning, since hormones produced by the thyroid are activated in the liver. Chief thyroid antagonists are the thymus, the pancreas, the parathyroid glands, and the hormones that nursing women's breasts produce during lactation.

Parathyroids

The parathyroids are four small glands, each about the size of a pea, that are attached to the thyroid gland. They regulate calcium levels in the blood even more strictly than the pancreas and adrenal glands regulate blood glucose. This regulatory function is lifesaving because proper blood calcium levels are essential for nerve transmission and muscle contraction; and, of course, the most important nerve transmissions and muscle contractions of all are those of the heart. The parathyroid gland must keep blood calcium levels high enough to feed the heart nerves and muscle. Then, if enough calcium is left over, the parathyroids can afford to make bone bank deposits. If blood calcium levels are too low, the parathyroids make withdrawals from the bone bank.

"The parathyroid gland is designed exclusively for calcium utilization; no other gland is dedicated to one mineral."[6] The parathyroid system operates so quickly that it can take calcium and phosphorus out of bones or deposit it back in a few fractions of a second.

The parathyroid glands produce a hormone that stimulates the bone marrow to carry out its various functions, including that of pro-ducing red blood cells. Nutritional support for the parathyroid allows it to release a hormone that stimulates bone bank deposits to be removed at a faster rate. In other words, it stimulates bone-destroying osteoclast cells.

While it may sound like a bad idea to stimulate cells that help break down bone, quite the opposite is true. In a healthy body with healthy bones, all aspects of the bone metabolic cycle are active. If any part of the bone-remodeling cycle is inactive or sluggish, the stage is set for unhealthy bones. An analogy brings home the point. Consider what would happen to a body that could ingest food but could not eliminate any of it. That's what happens to bones at the cellular level if the bone breakdown part of the cycle doesn't work.

The parathyroids back up their allies, the uterus or prostate, and cooperate with their friends: the pancreas, liver, and gonads. Their natural antagonist is the thyroid.

Adrenals

The adrenals are two triangular-shaped glands located one above each kidney. They make over thirty hormones that constantly shift to medi-ate differing stress levels. The adrenals play a central role in bone health because they participate in maintaining the correct mineral bal-ance. But when they are overactive, chronically turned on, they con-tinue to secrete stress hormones such as cortisol that, according to Susan Brown, Ph.D., "attach to bone cells and direct the withdrawal of calcium from the bones."[7] This is actually good for the body because this mechanism satisfies the high, short-term needs for calcium during stress. But the long-term effect of such adrenal stress hormone over-production is to thin bones.

That's not all. Under stress, adrenal hormones decrease calcium absorption in the intestines, and that, too, leads to increased withdrawal of calcium from the bone.[8] It's easy to tell when the adrenals are in a stress response because they secrete epinephrine (also called adrenalin). This hormone makes the heart race, the blood pressure elevate, arterioles constrict, digestion shut down, and glucose be liberated from the liver in preparation to fight, freeze, or flee.

Adrenals go into high gear under the influence of pain, fear, rage, or asphyxia (a state of suspended animation due to interference with the blood's oxygen supply). However, once such threats are over, the adrenals can forget to settle down, thus continuing to leach calcium deposits from the bone bank. That's one reason why it's so important not to live life on a constant adrenaline high. The invisible, bone-robbing cost of chronic stress can cause complete bone bank failure. One early symptom of adrenal weakening due to prolonged stress is that the body fills up with fluid. A warning sign of possible adrenal overload is puffy bags under the eyes.

Adrenals also produce other male-type sex hormones (including DHEA, or dehydroepiandrosterone, which is produced by the adrenal glands) that affect bone health positively. High DHEA levels are correlated with greater bone mineral content, and low levels with low bone mineral content. Therefore, keeping adrenals functioning well is one way to contribute to perfect bones.

But that's not the only reason to keep adrenals happy. Adrenals are the second backup to the heart after the thyroid. Also, they have some ability to compensate for low sex hormone levels if too little is secreted by the ovaries or testes. That is a major contribution to bone health, particularly after midlife.

Glands that cooperate with the adrenals include the thyroid, gonads, and pituitary. Those that antagonize adrenals are the pancreas, duodenum, thymus, gonads, and parathyroids.[9]

Gonads

Gonadal hormones play a key role in directing calcium metabolism for both women and men. Women's ovaries produce three types of gonadal hormones: estrogens, progesterone, and androgens. Estrogens have received a lot of attention for osteoporosis prevention because they increase calcium absorption and slow down or inhibit the rate of calcium withdrawal from the bone bank. However, the bone benefit of ingesting synthetic estrogen after menopause wanes after three to five years, John Lee, M.D., points out.[10] He concludes, "The strength of the estrogen-fixed mindset represents a victory of advertising over science."[11] Dr. Lee emphasizes that the crux of the problem is that "healthy, well nourished [ovarian] follicle cells produce a healthy balance of estrogen and progesterone." Malnourished follicles can shut down, requiring nutritional support to produce hormones. Well-nourished follicles (or the hormones they produce) are a necessary precondition for preventing or reversing osteoporosis. In men, the male sex hormone testosterone replaces estrogens and is produced by cells in the testes.

Progesterone is important to bone because it both stimulates the rate of bone bank deposits and helps limit withdrawals. As such, progesterone is possibly the most important hormone for healthy bones. A recent study in *The New England Journal of Medicine* reports that osteoporosis occurs in athletes to the degree that they become progesterone deficient. This hormone "acts directly on bone by engaging an osteoblast receptor or indirectly through competition for a glucocorticoid osteoblast receptor . . . the normal ovulatory cycle looks like a natural bone-activating, coherence cycle."[12] "Progesterone restores osteoblast function."[13]

Men's bodies also make progesterone, which the testes then turn into testosterone. Whether in men or women, according to John Lee, M.D., "Like progesterone, testosterone can stimulate new bone formation, increase bone density, and a lack of it can cause osteoporosis."[14] Men's hormone shifts are not as dramatic as women's during menopause, nonetheless, during men's corollary phase, sometimes called "andropause" or "viropause" or "manopause," testosterone levels do drop, also exposing men to the risks of developing sick bones. Restoring testosterone levels reverses these deleterious effects, even if they are a result of treatment with glucocorticoid drugs.[15]

Indeed, many people have inadequate or imbalanced levels of gonadal hormones. One reason is radiation, another is starvation. For example, people who keep themselves on a strict low-fat diet, with too few essential fatty acids, don't have enough of these building blocks to make sex hormones. Progesterone is formed predominantly in the ovaries to a lesser extent by the adrenals, and to some extent by nerves. It is formed in these tissues from cholesterol. Thus, people who suffer from anorexia also eventually stop producing the sex hormones necessary for bone health due to lack of these EFAs and other nutrients. Ultimately they become amenorrheic (without a period), and the longer they remain so, the more severely their bones are damaged. The same effect occurs in women who overexercise; their bones deteriorate when their bodies can no longer produce the sex hormones they need for bone health.

Another major contributor to gonadal hormone inadequacy is surgical removal of these hormone factories. Each year well over half a million women in the United States undergo surgical ovary removal, states Susan Brown, Ph.D.[16] "Thirty-four percent of U.S. women will have had their uterus removed by age 66. It's the second-most common surgery performed."[17] That translates to "650,000 or more hys-terectomies per year performed in the United States."[18] Of these, 1,200 die from the procedure.[19] In Britain, more than one thousand women per week (or fifty-two thousand per year) undergo hysterectomy, a surgery that contributes to loss of bone health and the onset of osteo-porosis.[20] Even when only the uterus is removed, the remaining ovaries often fail to function after the surgery.[21]

In terms of male hormones, states John Lee, M.D., "men castrated either surgically or chemically will experience accelerated osteoporo-sis within two to three years. Such a condition happens, for example, in the treatment of prostate cancer."[22] The current incidence of prostate cancer is one man in six. And the number one cancer among men between the ages of twenty and thirty-four is testicular cancer.[23]

Hypogonadal (low sex-hormone producing) men require sex hor-mone support to prevent osteoporosis for the same reasons that women require hormone replacement.[24] One key reason is that men will lose bone mass without sex hormone support. This support can easily be provided free of unwanted effects using the vegetarian sex hormone protocol (see below). Still, they are often denied it, the assumption being that higher testosterone levels are associated with greater risk of prostate cancer.

Whether in men, women, or children, evidence is mounting that estrogen becoming dominant over either progesterone or testosterone is dangerous to a number of bodily organs and processes. And this is true whether the dominance of estrogen is a result of estrogen pre-scription drugs or hormonal imbalances generated in the body itself. (See appendix III for a list of symptoms of estrogen dominance).

An often overlooked part of the reproductive hormonal system is the hormones that the mammary glands produce. Unfortunately, few studies have been conducted about their role. As far back as 1932, Henry Harrower, M.D., who wrote the seminal work of that time on the endocrine system, pointed out that the mammary glands secrete many substances science was not yet aware of.[25] Michael Dobbins, D.C., adds, "Many women's systems won't balance without adding mammary, which often acts as the catalyst to open up the [hormonal] system."[26]

Hypothalamus

The hypothalamus is a key regulatory player for all the members of the bone bank governing board. If the pituitary is the power on the throne, then the hypothalamus is the power behind the throne. It lies deep in the brain where it exerts control over the secretions of the other endocrine glands, especially stop and go messages to the nervous system. It even regulates the chair of the board, the pituitary. It also monitors sex hormone levels and their bodily effects. And it acts as a pacemaker to drive biological rhythms, including the sleep and wake cycle. John Lee, M.D., likens it to a giant analog computer complex that can make and send signals to the pituitary gland. The hypothalamus can control the autonomic (involuntary) nervous system balance and modulate the immune system. It even influences emotional states and the responses that the body makes to them.

The hypothalamus gland's functions are influenced by pain and by smell, by digestive functions in the intestines, and by concentrations of nutrients, electrolytes, water, and hormones. It also responds to messages from the limbic, or emotional, brain. This input into the endocrine system by the nervous system is one of the reasons all the hormonal regulators in action are referred to as "neuroendocrine function."

Hypothalamic operations are interfered with by stress, especially emotional pressure, and by poor diet, especially protein deficiency and pollutants, including synthetic Progestins and birth control pills. Such deficiencies and pollutants, says John Lee, M.D., create hypothalamic imbalances that can lead to "decreased immune response, decreased adrenal response, sleep disorders, peptic ulcers, depression, anxiety, panic, rage, learning disorders, and hormone disorders."[27] The hypothalamus's functions can be brought into check by two of its main antagonists: neurotransmitters and pituitary feedback.

Hormones play a critical role in bone health. How might hormonal imbalances affect someone? John G., an eighty-one-year-old grandfather, reports, "When I was seventy-five, I had some symptoms, including loss of bladder control. I went to the doctor and found out I had prostate cancer. First I had radiation for several months. Then I began to complain about my hip. So they took an X-ray and found out that the cancer was metastasized to the bone. The doctor decided that my cancer was feeding on testosterone, so [to get rid of the testosterone] I was given a choice of a chemical or surgical approach. I chose surgical, a total orchiectomy, complete removal of the testicles. I didn't like the odds for the chemical approach: fifteen months to live."

He continues, "Then I became interested in an alternative approach. A New York doctor wrote a book about macrobiotics, and I started [reading] it right after I recovered from surgery. Because they'd given me sixteen months to live after the surgery, my daughter suggested that I get tested. I got tested by Mary Jane Mack, R.N. I went on the protocols for yeast and virus. I took the protocols, and in two and a quarter months happened to have another appointment back with the urologist. After doing some tests, he came back in shock; my PSA [prostate-specific antibody] level had dropped to zero. I talked with the doctors about these alternatives, but they took the position that there was nothing in their medical practice that would lead to recommending it, but since it was an alternative practice, try it. Then when I got the wonderful test results, the doctor wouldn't admit it was from the muscle testing and clinical nutrition. But I thought it was. That was three years ago, and I've had two zero PSAs since."

Since the surgery, John says he's "developed a stoop and am shrinking in height. I can't drink out of a normal cup for coffee because my head tilts too far forward. I have to put my head way back. I've had muscle tension a long time. I was once evaluated by a psychiatrist; his conclusion was I had a psychoneurosis tension state. I had no muscle problems until I got my sciatic condition. In my right leg I have to be very careful in how I move my leg a certain way; I get the feeling of precramping." He's also noticed tooth pain. He feels that "the stoop and losing height happened some before the surgery, but after it happened much faster. I'm eighty-one years and a quarter now; I was seventy-eight when I had the surgery."

He continues, "I haven't taken any hormones after the surgery. I talked to my urologist about some chemical replacement, and he said he preferred I not take any out of concern I might have a flare-up. I'd had bone cancer at the time of the operation. I'd prefer to have some sort of treatment or replacement of testosterone lost by surgery. I have so much fatigue, and that's very limiting. I need morning naps and afternoon naps and naps before bed. I also have a softening of my muscular structure. I don't believe I increased breast size but I got a lot flabbier. Then, two years ago, I started to have symptoms of Parkinson's."

I tested John during our interview and found that his osteoporosis reflex did indeed test weak, and also that he was very weak for sex hormone protocols and oils. Despite his PSAs staying so low and his symptoms of osteoporosis, his urologist has not recommended any hormone replacement. However, with the last exam, John reports, his urologist finally "recommended a diet that included low fat and soy and a lot of what's recommended by macrobiotics. He even said he's on it himself."

John clearly demonstrates a need for the concentrated nutritional protocols that would support his hormonal system. However, the form of nutritional support needed to help restore hormonal balance is highly individual. John needs sex hormone support and essential fatty acids. Maureen Schaub decided to find out what she needed.

Maureen, a beautician and the mother of two children, already had a dowager's hump and back pain at age thirty-three. She says, "I was worried about not getting enough calcium, and my back was hurting. I got inflamed discs a lot in my upper back, which I think is due to the stress of my profession, having my arms up all the time. My grandma on my dad's side had osteoporosis, and that's always concerned me. Even before my profession, I was hunched over. I am intolerant both to lactose and milk protein; my digestive system is very sensitive. The older I get, the more back problems I have. Also my energy level wasn't good, so I decided to give this muscle testing and clinical nutrition a try and see what it could do with me.

"First I had an infection in one of my lungs from my work environment, all the chemicals I'd been around, so I took Parotid PMG [SP; see chapter 11]. I still take a low maintenance dose based on the amount of chemicals I'm around all day."

Such chemicals can indeed deplete bone bank deposits. Even more significant is her need for various forms of hormonal support. The first of these was her thyroid, for which she took Thytrophin PMG (SP) and Organic Iodine (SP). She explains, "I started having thyroid problems when I was thirteen. My thyroid was so enlarged it came out to where my chin is. The doctor sent me to a thyroid specialist. He wanted my body to try to develop on its own, so he didn't give me anything. So I took kelp on my own. I don't know if it helped or not. When I had my first child, my daughter, my thyroid whacked out." She was given diethylstilbestrol (DES) to guarantee that she wouldn't miscarry. She adds, "My mom took DES, too, to guarantee that she wouldn't miscarry me." DES is a potent synthetic estrogen given to two to six million women to prevent miscarriage, resulting in increased risk of clear cell adenocarcinoma of the vagina and cervix in their daughters.[28]

Thyroid support was central to restoring Maureen's hormonal balance in preparation for bone repair. But three other hormone factories needed nutrition too, probably due to trying to back up a weak thyroid all those years. Over time, she has also needed support for: her pituitary, for which she has taken either Pituitrophin PMG (SP) or Symplex F; her sex hormones, for which she took Ovex and Catalyn; and her adrenals, for which she took B_6-Niacinamide (SP).

After her hormone system was back in balance, Maureen began addressing nutritional needs for bone repair. She needed a blood builder, for which she took e-Poise. She also needed gallbladder support, and she was put on Betafood. Then, she says,

> I was taking Calcium Lactate [to supplement her calcium intake], but I would still hold my body tense. So Laura [her practitioner] put me on Cal-Ma Plus [calcium lactate plus parathyroid support] and also the flaxseed pill [Linum B_6, SP] to help it absorb better. I started noticing a difference within a week, especially my shoulder area and back, being able to relax better. And the pain subsided. I still take it, and feel like I'll take it forever. I'd rather, knowing I don't use dairy products. I want to make sure I'm in better health.
>
> Since I've been on the Cal-Ma Plus, my discs inflame far less often, and far less severely when they do. Before, my discs would be inflamed quite often, but now it's only during the times I'm really busy at work. If I don't take the flaxseed oil with it, I do notice a difference . . . a little stiffer feeling. The oil helps it get into the system better. I took three Cal-Ma Plus a day orig-

inally, and now take two or three each night. If I go totally off it, if I forget, I feel the difference in my body. I've been taking it now for four months.

Now I give my kids flaxseed oil and calcium lactate when they have growing pains, and it takes the growing pains away. Their bones are growing so fast. Doing it the natural way is so much better than man-made drugs that suppress the problem. The clinical nutrition gets to the core of the problem, which is important to me.[29]

RESTORING HORMONAL BALANCE

The following hormonal products help feed the body so it can make its own hormones and bring them into balance. Vegetarian products (other than herbs) for all the various hormone systems are built around providing essential fatty acid precursors; therefore, products for general hormonal support as well as for pituitary, ovarian, uterine, testicular, prostatic, and mammary hormones are similar.

Herbal hormonal tonics help normalize or balance levels of estrogen and other hormones, according to herbalist and author Amanda McQuade Crawford, "by affecting the feedback regulation of the endocrine system, assisting natural functioning and reversing infertility, irregular menstrual cycles, and the effects of the birth-control pill."[30] These include: sarsaparilla root, red clover flower, black cohosh root, *Vitex* (chaste tree), dong quai, and saw palmetto. All are described in this book.

Protocols are made from a combination of products as determined by your health practitioner. In the product descriptions below, "SP" designates Standard Process formulations, and "MH" designates those made by MediHerb. The sources for herbal information are *Principles and Practice of Phytotherapy: Modern Herbal Medicine,* by Simon Mills and Kerry Bone, and *MediHerb Innovative Herbal Solutions Product Catalog 2001,* unless otherwise noted. All products mentioned but not described here are detailed in other chapters (see index).

Whole Food Concentrates for Pituitary Support

Catalyn (SP) was the first product that Royal Lee made when he started Standard Process. His chief goal was to provide nutritional support for all the endocrine glands. Catalyn acts as a biochemical catalyst. It contains a myriad of vitamins, trace minerals, and enzymes. (See also chapter 7.)

E-Manganese (SP) supports the anterior pituitary's high demand for manganese and vitamin E complex.

For-Til B$_{12}$ (SP) is often recommended for hormone support because it is rich in vitamin E and other factors needed to make sex hormones. It contains tillandsia, found in Spanish moss. It is excellent for people who are fatigued and worn out.[31]

Pituitrophin PMG (SP) is used for general pituitary support and when the pituitary is hyperactive (hyperpituitary). It supports people with metabolic disorders, delayed healing, gastrointestinal ulcers, and nervous symptoms. It is high in trace minerals, B$_{12}$, and vitamin E complex. It is combined with Neuroplex and E-Manganese (see above) for a weak or low functioning gland (hypopituitary).

Symplex F (female) or **Symplex M** (male) (SP) is indicated for multiple hormone imbalances, including hypothalamic imbalances. These products contain nutrition that supports the pituitary, thyroid, adrenals, and ovaries or testes. It also contains chlorophyll (see chapter 8). It may especially be needed after the hormonal shifts of menopause or prepuberty. Because pituitary support can help balance the entire hormonal system, Symplex F or M can benefit the bone bank in all the ways discussed above. An additional advantage is that it can help balance mood swings, and it may improve sexual responsiveness in both men and women. Many practitioners are also using it to support brain growth and functioning in children, including those with cerebral palsy and/or mental retardation.

Whole Food Concentrates for Thyroid Support

A-C Carbamide (SP, vegetarian) supports the thyroid function having to do with the osmotic transfer of body fluids through cell walls; therefore, it is used for water-retention problems related to low thyroid function. (See chapter 10.)

Iodomere (SP) is also a source of protein-bound iodine in combination with sea minerals. It contains portions of sea conch. It gives nutritional support to a sluggish thyroid, especially when low thyroid function is associated with fluid retention, which results in swelling and wastes backing up in the kidneys.

Min-Tran (SP, vegetarian), short for "mineral tranquilizers," provides a source of alkaline ash minerals combined with calcium lactate. These are nutrients that support thyroid T_1 function. They are sometimes recommended for people who are very tired until their tiredness is gone.

Organic Iodine (SP, vegetarian) supports the thyroid by providing protein-bound iodine. It is used to control hot flashes in menopausal women.

Organic Minerals (SP, vegetarian) are a different blend of minerals also used for thyroid support. (See chapter 7.)

Thytrophin PMG (SP) contains a combination of nutrition designed to provide general support to the thyroid gland. If the thyroid is overworking, Antronex may be added. Also, Thytrophin PMG may be combined with Allorganic Trace Minerals B_{12} to support slowing the thyroid.[32] If the thyroid is underproducing, Betafood and Niacinamide B_6 may be added.

Vegetarian whole food concentrate products for thyroid support are often chosen from the following: T_1: Min-Tran; T_4: Organic Minerals; Organic Iodine; Linum B_6; Chlorophyll; RNA; T_4: Organic Iodine; Linum B_6; Chlorophyll Complex; and T_3: A-C Carbamide. All herbal products given below are vegetarian.

Herbal Products for Thyroid Support

Bladderwrack (MH) contains iodine to promote thyroid health. It is used in cases of low thyroid functioning. It is rich in trace minerals, and it is also used to aid a sluggish digestion. (For this function, see also chapter 10.)

Bugleweed (MH) is used to rebalance an overactive thyroid gland. It contains phenolics, flavonoids, and other compounds that, together, support healthy metabolism.

Coleus (MH) is also used to improve low thyroid functioning. It increases levels of cAMP, a bodily compound that is required to support thyroid stimulating hormone (TSH).

Lemon Balm (MH) is often used when a hyperthyroid condition is related to environmental and nervous system stresses. It calms the thyroid by way of an essential oil consisting of a large number of monoterpenes and sesquiterpenes.

Motherwort (MH) calms a hyperactive thyroid via the nervous system and also supports female reproductive system health. Therefore it is often recommended when both systems are in need of support.

Rehmannia Complex (MH) is a liquid formulation containing *Rehmannia, Bupleurum, Hemidesmus,* and feverfew. They support healthy adrenal gland and liver health and support the body's natural defenses against environmental stress. This combination is particularly useful if the thyroid is hyperactive due to an autoimmune component.

Whole Food Concentrates for Parathyroid Support

Cal-Ma Plus (SP) contains Calcium Lactate combined with desiccated parathyroid gland to enhance the absorption of calcium. Desiccated products are made from a concentrate of the whole gland. Cal-Ma Plus is designed specifically for parathyroid support. Desiccated Parathyroid (SP) draws calcium from the reserves and puts it in the blood. Supporting the parathyroid gland can sometimes unlock the door to healing bones. Cal-Ma Plus is also used when the body is unable to metabolize iron. If the parathyroid is underactive, Cal-Ma Plus may be combined with Cataplex F. If the parathyroid is overactive, Cataplex D may be substituted for the Cataplex F.[33]

Cataplex D (SP) is used to balance an overactive parathyroid gland (hyperparathyroid). It is rarely needed, as most people have enough vitamin D in their diets or make sufficient quantities by exposure to sunlight.

Cataplex F (SP) is also used for parathyroid support. Men with prostate problems or women with uterine problems, whether these organs have been removed or irradiated, sometimes need to address parathyroid gland nutrition with F Perles because the parathyroid gland backs up the uterus or prostate. Cataplex F supports the parathyroid gland in producing parathyroid hormone. Cataplex F is also used to calm down the thyroid because it contains unsaturated fatty acids that make iodine more diffusible, available for use by the thyroid so it can balance itself. (See the previous chapter for more on essential fatty acids.)

Whole Food Concentrates for Adrenal Support

One of the symptoms of weak adrenal glands is a low level of DHEA (short for dehydroepiandrosterone), a hormone produced naturally by the adrenal glands and also by the ovaries. Some studies have concluded that DHEA increases bone strength. Therefore it has been recommended as part of the treatment for osteoporosis. Alan Gaby, M.D., explains that DHEA is the only hormone that appears capable of both inhibiting bone bank withdrawals (bone resorption) and stimulating bone bank deposits, or bone formation. High DHEA levels are associated with higher density of the spinal bones. Women with osteoporosis have been shown to have lower levels of DHEA at all ages than women without osteoporosis.[34]

However, Bruce West, D.C., cautions, "dabbling in hormones has a cascade effect . . . you are being sold a hormone product that simply masks a laboratory finding of low DHEA levels. And worse, it leaves the more serious condition developing and tinkers with the balance of your adrenal gland hormones. . . . Don't complicate matters by taking DHEA supplements."[35] He adds that since DHEA can be converted into estrogen and testosterone in the body, it may be "the kiss of death" for a woman prone to estrogen-induced cancer or a man prone to testosterone-induced cancer of the prostate.[36] Michael Dobbins, D.C., concurs: "For DHEA, if you need it, make it; don't buy it. Support your adrenals. Feed them. Low DHEA is adrenal insufficiency."[37]

B$_6$ Niacinamide (SP) contains adrenal hormone precursors that support the bone bank. It also contains nutrients central to making connective tissue. Michael Dobbins, D.C., explains that proteins and trace minerals bind to the organic collagen net. Vitamin B$_6$ greatly aids production of these proteins.[38] Niacinamide is used as nutritional support for adrenal insufficiency.

Catechol (North American Pharmacal) is a stress relief balancer that is recommended for blood types O and AB.

Cortiguard (North American Pharmacal, vegetarian) is used to buffer the adverse effects of the cortisol released during stress. It is particularly recommended for blood types A and B.

Drenamin (SP) is a combination of nutrients that supports weak adrenal glands. Because it is made from animal adrenal glands, it may be recommended for people whose adrenals are chronically fatigued, for those who have low blood sugar, and for those who crave salt. Drenamin functions as a quick-start spark for people with acute adrenal exhaustion.

Drenatrophin PMG (SP) contains the nutritional substrate that adrenal glands need for repair. It is often recommended for people with weak adrenals who demonstrate respiratory weaknesses or allergies.

Whole Desiccated Adrenal (SP) is often used short-term when rapid adrenal support is needed, as in shock or sudden severe stress. It may be used for two or three weeks, but not long-term.[39] Its use is not recommended for more than thirty days.[40]

Vegetarian adrenal support usually combines Black Currant Seed Oil and Chlorophyll Complex.

Herbal Products for Adrenal Support

Ashwaganda or **Withania Somnifera** (MH) is a liquid extract containing various compounds that have a tonic and adaptogenic effect for the entire body. It encourages healthy responses to environmental stresses and also supports bones by promoting normal blood production.

Licorice (MH) is a liquid extract that's an excellent adrenal tonic, but it is for short-term use only. That's because its aldosterone-like effects may cause fluid retention and possibly elevate blood pressure over time. It also supports healthy lung function, facilitates the body's natural ability to break up respiratory secretions, and encourages normal bowel movements.

Rehmannia (MH) is a liquid extract that serves as an excellent tonic to support the adrenals. It has the advantage of being safe to use when blood pressure concerns are present. It aids the body's normal responses to occasional stress, including environmental stress. And because of the adrenals' role in governing body fluids, it encourages normal fluid elimination.

Siberian Ginseng (MH) is a liquid extract rich in compounds that enhance the body's natural ability to adapt to temporary stress. It supports physical and mental endurance, promotes vitality, restores and enhances immune system function, and acts as a general tonic.

Withania Complex (MH) is a liquid formulation containing a combination of licorice, ashwaganda, skullcap, and Korean ginseng. Together they act as synergists to provide a powerful tonic to the entire body and assist it in adapting to the changes and stresses of everyday life, including supporting the body's natural defenses against emotional and environmental stressors.

Nettle leaf, sarsaparilla, and devil's club are also sometimes used to support the adrenal glands in particular and the endocrines in general.[41]

Whole Food Concentrates for Gonadal Support

The following are concentrated nutritional protocols that, according to Mary Jane Mack, R.N., "work at a deeper level than hormone creams" (described below).[42] They provide the nutritional support to organs so they can manufacture their own progesterone.

Orchex (SP) provides nutritional support for the production and balance of sex hormones. It is used in acute situations for people whose hormone production is so far off balance that they're about to blow their stack. It's also given to women for menopausal hypertension and to men with hypertension.[43]

Ovex (SP) supports female androgen production. It aids calcium assimilation, supports the ovaries, and provides vitamin E for steroid hormone production. It was developed to stop heavy menstrual bleeding. It contains enzymes that help the body make progesterone instead of estrogen. When progesterone levels are too low, periods last too long; in an estrogen deficiency, periods are too short.[44] Ovex has demonstrated good clinical results in women who had difficulty getting pregnant or who have hot flashes, PMS, or depression, as it supports weak ovaries.

Prost-X (SP) is an aqueous prostate extract that helps transport calcium into bones. If the prostate lacks calcium, it will become enlarged.[45]

Utrophin PMG (SP) is an extract that promotes healthy tissue and balances hormone production and its storage in the uterus.[46] Some practitioners have reported that this product (or, for men, Prost-X) can have an antidepressant effect similar to Prozac, which is a drug that also works on the hormonal system. "The drug masks what's really going on," states Mary Jane Mack, R.N.; "it takes care of superficial pain or discomfort but underneath is still the same problem."[47]

Herbal Products for Gonadal Support

Black Cohosh (MH) is a liquid extract that eases the effects of menopause and menstruation, promotes the body's normal resistance function, and helps maintain and support healthy joints.

Chaste Tree (MH) is a tablet that contains an essential oil and flavo-noids that help promote a natural, healthy balance within the female endocrine system, supporting female reproductive system health, and easing temporary feelings of tension associated with the menstrual cycle. There are no herbs that are progesterogenic in nature; however, chaste tree, also called *Vitex*, does promote the body's production of progesterone. It acts to improve the integrity of the corpus luteum (the part of the ovary that produces progesterone) while it is developing in the follicular phase of the menstrual cycle.

Korean Ginseng (MH) promotes vitality and stamina, works as a tonic, supports and maintains cellular health, enhances mental clarity, and supports the body's natural defenses against emotional and environ-mental stressors.

Phytoestrogens are a group of compounds found in plants that can influence the body's estrogen activity. These compounds may either provide precursors so the body can manufacture its own estrogen or act as a weak estrogen. Hundreds of plants contain these compounds, including red clover, licorice, dong quai, soy beans, flaxseeds, black cohosh, and alfalfa. Animals have been known to graze selectively on these plants to enhance or diminish fertility.[48] Phytoestrogens are a relatively safe way to affect estrogen activity in the body.

Sage (MH) is a liquid extract that provides relief from discomfort asso-ciated with menopause. It is a central nervous system stimulant. It also eases the effects of intestinal gas buildup and supports oral health.

Wild Yam (MH) is a liquid extract made from the root and the rhizome of the wild yam. There is something about wild yam that has an osteogenic effect. It contains a variety of compounds, including dioscin, that together ease the effects of symptoms associated with menopause. It also provides antispasmodic activity to ease occasional spasms of smooth muscle, including those associated with the menstrual cycle.

Wild Yam Complex (MH) tablets contain wild yam, other estrogen-promoting herbs (false unicorn, sage, and Korean ginseng), plus St. John's wort. It can help provide relief from discomfort associated with menopause, balance and support normal female physiology and function, calm the nerves, restore balance in temporary mood swings, and provide antispasmodic activity.

Sex hormones such as those for progesterone and testosterone aid new bone formation equally. Some sex hormone products are synthetic and carry the risks associated with their respective oral hormone replacement product (see chapter 3). In addition, it is difficult to regulate their levels, and the hormonal system can become severely unbalanced. Therefore, many health practitioners recommend natural products that are bio-identical or that contain hormone precursors so that the body can make the amount of hormone it needs with no side effects.

Recently, three creams have become available. Their purpose is to provide either the hormones themselves or the building blocks to help the body make its own hormones.The first of these is testosterone propionate ointment cream, obtainable as a prescription formulated by a pharmacy. It provides testosterone when levels are low.

The second cream is phytoestrogen cream. It contains a variety of herbs with plant compounds that are structurally similar to estrogen and thus may help to relieve symptoms of estrogen imbalance without the side effects often caused by synthetic estrogens.[49]

The third cream is natural progesterone cream made from Mexican yams. Science has known about this source of natural progesterone since 1949.[50] This natural product has been shown to completely halt women's osteoporosis in its tracks, reversing bone bank withdrawals and restoring bone without the dangerous side effects of synthetic Progestins. Progesterone cream has also had encouraging results with men (progesterone is converted to testosterone in the liver when the body needs it), but has not yet been scientifically studied.[51] Progesterone cream is especially used for follicular inadequacy (when the ovarian follicle doesn't produce enough progesterone). The answer to this condition, John Lee, M.D., states, "is good nutrition, avoidance of toxins, and proper supplementation, when indicated for hormone balance, or real, honest-to-God, natural progesterone."[52] Lee adds, "It is a mystery to me why synthetic Progestins are recommended when the natural progesterone is available, cheaper and safer."[53]

Whole Food Concentrates for Hypothalamic Support

Hypothalamus PMG (SP) is often recommended when hormonal imbalance is accompanied by depression and disturbances in the thirst and satiation centers. It's for people who say, "I don't get satisfied! I eat a meal and still want to continue eating."[54]

Neuroplex provides nutritional support for the hypothalamus so it can coordinate the activity of the endocrine system with that of the nervous system. It is also used to support people with brain stem injury, children who can't talk, stutterers, and individuals with autism—any situation in which there is evidence of difficulty processing thoughts, with flow of information. Neuroplex is also used for people with spinal cord injuries.

Symplex F or **Symplex M** and **For-Til B$_{12}$** are also used for nutritional support for the hypothalamus (see above).

Balancing the hormonal system has a variety of effects, depending on the person. For people who are devoid of the food precursors necessary to guard the hormones from oxidation, a fatty acid imbalance may next be revealed (Point Three). Maureen Schaub's next layer of healing dealt with minerals (Point Two). On the other hand, Mary Jane Mack, R.N., notes, "It can go back to blood quality [lack of nutrition in the blood, see Point Six] because the body has nothing to work with."[55]

For me, getting my hormones balanced opened the floodgates to allow mineral deposits to return to my bone bank. That proved to be the last crucial link in creating abundant mineral deposits in my bone bank. The minerals poured back into my bones, and I could feel my strength returning, not weekly or daily, but hourly. My bones were healing so rapidly now that I had to carry minerals with me and take them throughout the day to meet the demand. But it was worth it. I became able to sit, to carry things, to move swiftly. And I developed stamina. Instead of dragging, my body demanded to be active and to move, a subject of the next chapter.

TEN

Stimulating Deposit Activity: Muscles and Metabolism

ACTIVITY IS THE VERY ESSENCE OF LIFE. Because bones are living tissue, to stay healthy, they require both voluntary, energetic movement and the involuntary movements of the metabolic cycle. Voluntary activities create demand, which stimulates bones to respond. Exercise both activates the bone bank deposit process (because bone-building osteoclast cells increase their activity) and reduces bone bank withdrawals (because the bone-destroying cells slow their activity). This state of affairs—receiving lots of deposits and reducing withdrawals—is indeed a happy one for bones.

Without the catalyst of exercise, bones become weak. When bones are at rest, as when they are in a cast, they are protected from mechanical stress. The bones become weaker, decreasing in mass. When removed from the cast, they respond to additional stresses and will again remodel and increase strength until they return to normal.

The rapid decrease in bone mass that results from immobilization is a long-known fact. It's been especially well documented in people requiring bed rest and those with some regional form of immobilization such as partial or total paralysis. In fact, people who don't move are in danger of having their mineral deposits made not in their bones but in their soft tissues, such as arteries, or formed into stones that can lodge in the kidneys.[1]

Gravity is essential to keeping bones healthy. Astronauts in outer space lose bone mass, not because of immobilization, but because of lack of gravity. The Skylab astronauts, for example, stayed highly active but still withstood bone losses comparable to bedridden people. In a weightless environment, their bones didn't have the demand that carrying their own body weight creates on earth to keep them healthy.[2]

VOLUNTARY MOVEMENT

Exercise promotes healthy bones because, biochemically, the bones require calcium in response to bearing weight. When backpacking, for example, bones undergo the mechanical stress of the load they're carrying, which stimulates bone bank deposit activity (osteoblasts). It is likely that hormones (in particular, somatotropin) give the marching orders to these bone-building cells. This means that putting demands on the skeleton via exercise is a nonnegotiable part of the quest for perfect bones.

Kinds of Exercise

No doubt, any movement is better than none. Studies have demonstrated that some non-weight-bearing exercises may be helpful to bones. But not all exercise is equal in building bone mass. The most effective bone-health-promoting activities are those that make muscles work against gravity or resistance: aerobic, weight-bearing, and resistance exercises. As Clare Dover states, "Pulling of the muscles on the skeleton through exercise and activity keeps the skeleton strong and the bone responsive to the message to rebuild properly."[3]

For example, people who play tennis have heavier bones in the arm they use to serve the ball than in their non-serving arm. And long-distance runners' spines are more substantial than those of people who rarely exercise, Clare Dover points out.[4] "Bone tissue is dynamic and, as it is worked, it increases its absorption of the minerals that give it density."[5]

As part of its osteoporosis prevention project, the Colorado Department of Health recommends the following activities as best for bones: walking, stair climbing, hiking, jogging, skiing, cross-country ski machines, stair-step machines, dancing, aerobic dancing, treadmill walking, weight training, tennis, step classes, and gardening. The department adds that "swimming or bicycling are probably also helpful, especially when swimmers use fins and paddles, and bicyclers ride up hills." They conclude that "it is important to exercise both the upper and lower parts of the body to strengthen all of the bones."[6]

If you like to swim and want to keep that as your primary bone-building activity, you might be interested in the results of the broadest study done yet about bone density, conducted at Australia's Edith Cowan University. "Doctors surveyed 60 female athletes and found that those who had engaged in high-impact sports for 20–30 years had much stronger bones than those who swam."[7] These findings imply that swimmers in their twenties and thirties might want to start introducing some weight-bearing activity into their exercise programs.

According to some experts, the static, slow hatha yoga stretching exercises that include resistance can strengthen bones. This is true in part because weight-bearing exercises encourage calcium and silicon deposits in bones, helping to strengthen them. According to yoga instructor Christina Brown, the asana practices of hatha yoga encourage nutrient supply to the bones in general. Hatha yoga also has the advantage of offering many postures that allow the upper body to bear weight, thus strengthening bones in the arms, wrists, and cervical vertebrae. Additionally, inverted yoga postures can help balance hormones, in part through increasing blood supply to relevant endocrine glands. The shoulder stand and plow poses in particular encourage blood supply to the throat, the location of the parathyroid gland. This gland produces a hormone that affects calcium levels in the bone, and helps find an optimum balance between the breaking down of old bone, laying down of new bone, and bone remineralization. Yoga breathing and deep relaxation also rebalance the body via the nervous system.[8]

Physical therapist Julie Jacobs, of Seattle, Washington, says that weight-bearing and repetitive exercise are limited methods for strengthening bone. Because healthy bones need to be not only strong but also supple and resilient, she teaches classes called "Continuum Movement," which include breath, sound, and movement to awaken bone's inherent adaptability and resilience.[9]

Currently, research is being conducted on the effects of an experimental osteoporosis-fighting machine that applies electric and magnetic fields (EMFs) to bones. The person stands on a vibrating platform that sends a gentle buzz through every bone in their body.[10]

Since magnetic fields are catalysts to the body's chemical reactions, magnetic devices are also being investigated for their effect on bone. For example, Dr. Dean Bonlie has been investigating magnetism since he found relief from arthritic back pain using a magnetic sleep pad that he designed to create a negatively charged magnetic field. Studies on the pad's effect on bone are just beginning, but a nationally recognized researcher reported that her bone mineral density increased from −1.8 to +4.8 (negative numbers indicate problems either present or developing; positive numbers indicate healthy bones). She is now conducting a pilot study on the effect of magnetism on osteoporosis. Meanwhile, it is postulated that magnetism improves oxygen-carrying capacity, assimilation of nutrients, manufacture of enzymes, metabolic waste removal, reduction of free radicals, and tissue regeneration and healing.[11]

Last is a simple but often-overlooked fact not emphasized sufficiently in the literature on building bone: rest and sleep are required to build bone. No matter how much you exercise and how well, the body only builds bone during sleep. Therefore, many practitioners recommend taking certain hormone-supporting and bone-supporting protocols immediately before going to bed. That way the supplies for building bone and the hormonal orders to build it are both present and can go into action while the body is in deep relaxation and rest.

Who Can Benefit?

To reap the bone benefits of exercise, apparently the best course of action would be to have been active in childhood, before age twenty, when most peak bone mass develops. For example, of 155 women studied in Bath, England, those who "recalled doing a great deal of walking when they were youngsters had developed the strongest thigh bones," which are the strongest bones in the body.[12]

But if you led a sedentary childhood, and even a sedentary adulthood up to this point, don't despair. It's never too late to reap the benefits of activity. Indeed, exercise all through life is an important tool to prevent osteoporosis. Men and women age fifty to seventy who exercise regularly have been shown to have 30 percent denser bones than their nonexercising counterparts. How, then, to begin?

Beginning Safely

Weight-bearing exercise provides an important benefit to bones, but it may be more than many osteoporosis sufferers can manage. That was true for me at the low point of my bone loss. At first I couldn't even walk because I would become injured and have to spend a long, inactive time recovering. Yet I knew that becoming active was essential. Luckily my health care professionals advised me to stay below my expectations; in other words, to proceed, but not to push myself. The key for my beginning to exercise safely was getting into water, where I could move slowly and carefully with the water supporting me.

From there, I slowly graduated to being able to walk, then carry a backpack, then hike, bike, and use weights. Gradually, my body relearned to be active.

If you are fairly inactive now, you may feel defeated if you think you have to do thirty to forty-five minutes of aerobic activity nearly every day, as many experts recommend. If that goal sounds impossible, you may want to start with the aim of increasing what you now do. After all, your body wants to move—that's how it is designed.

Grown-ups have to exert a lot of effort to get kids to sit still. Being in motion is the natural state of the body, and a healthy body continues to want activity. If supported properly with good nutrition, healthy activity, and plenty of sleep, it will slowly regain its ability to do all kinds of things. Eventually your body can return to that free, childlike state, when you want to move and can do so joyfully.

To get to that state of recovery, Barbara Drinkwater, an exercise physiologist and one of the country's leading bone density experts, recommends that you increase the duration and intensity of your exercise regimen by no more than 10 percent per week.[13]

Don't be stymied by not knowing which activity you should do. Think about what your body is currently able to do and what would be fun. Anything is better than nothing. Do something, if only for two minutes. Then congratulate yourself for it. Refuse to allow room for a negative turn of mind. Don't measure what you did against anyone else, or even against your ultimate goal. If you moved more today than yesterday, you're improving already. Now focus on what you can do tomorrow.

If you have trouble exercising because your physical condition is too deteriorated, then follow the same developmental stages that your bones did embryonically. Get into some water. Start by moving your arms and legs in a warm bath, if necessary, and when you can do that, proceed to a warm hot tub or pool. Next add weight resistance while still exercising in the water. From there you'll eventually progress to being able to perform strenuous movement on land. You'll be moving back up the phylogenetic scale, from jellyfish to human!

Remember that swimming, although it is a good place to start, has less benefit for bones than weight-bearing activities. So, as soon as you can do so safely, include some walking. Later you can add biking or even jogging or aerobics. Playing tennis, basketball, jumping on a trampoline, jumping rope, and weight lifting are beneficial too.

The key to reaping the benefits of exercise is to build it into your daily routine and to have fun. If you use an appointment book or calendar, make an appointment with yourself, and then exercise during that time. If that's too big a step, then use that appointment time to shape a plan and decide what's possible for you.

Since it's easy to exercise the jaw muscle, you could even begin by talking with someone about your exercise goals and ask for their ideas and support. Start by checking in with your health care provider to assess your current fitness level and to find out what a realistic beginning step might be for you. Then you might meet with a staff member at a health and fitness club. If talking is your favorite activity, then combine a fitness activity with visits with friends. Take a walk, swim, or visit a health or fitness club together.

Some people keep their bones strong because their job involves physical labor. If your job is sedentary, consider a hobby that involves physical work, like gardening or taking care of horses. That will make it easy for you to stay motivated. You don't have to spend money on a hobby or a health club. Walking is the easiest weight-bearing exercise; it costs nothing, requires no special equipment, and provides marvelous benefits for bones.

How Often?

Once you have selected your bone-building activities, how often should you do them for maximum bone bank benefit? For aerobic, weight-bearing activity, most sources recommend a minimum of three twenty- to thirty-minute sessions per week. For strength training, dietician Sharon Bortz, M.S., R.D., reports excellent effects from strength training only two days a week. In a study she worked on at the Human Nutrition Research Center on Aging at Tufts University in Boston, she reported, "The women started with a 5-minute warm-up of light aerobic activity . . . then performed two sets of eight repetitions. The resistance was set at levels that did not allow them to do more than eight reps. Once they could do more, the resistance was increased." The study emphasized working the muscles "most used for activities of daily living; namely the knee extension, double leg press, lateral pull down, back extension, and the abdominal curl." Apparently these activities work because "muscle mass is directly related to strength and strength is related to bone mass."[14]

Such aerobic, weight-bearing activities and resistance exercises also have been shown to build bone mass in men. "Men who reported regular exercise had significantly higher BMD (bone mineral density) at the spine and hip," according to the *Journal of Bone Mineral Research*.[15]

Whether your activity is aerobic or resistance exercise, include some stretches in your routine. Always stretch after your muscles are warmed up. And remember, your body needs time to build up. Slow and steady wins the race. One physician tells his patients, "It takes time for this process to occur, therefore you don't want to increase stresses too fast—that will make a stress fracture. Therefore, build up slowly when exercising."[16]

However, too much of a good thing is no longer a good thing, so don't overdo it. Bad bones can happen to good people when they get more exercise than their hormonal systems can handle. Overly reducing body fat results in low hormone production, and these are key factors in the setup for osteoporosis. Studies show that problems with bone loss develop when levels of physical activity are so high that they are associated with impaired ovulation (see chapter 9).[17] If you try to make exercise the only part of what you do to prevent osteoporosis, you could be very sorry.

Carol Gieg (whom we met in chapters 1 and 2) exercised constantly from childhood on. She walked, she hiked, she biked, she went kayaking, and so forth. If exercise were the only answer to bone health, she should have had fabulous, perfect bones. Instead, she has had numerous stress fractures and severe osteoporosis, as demonstrated in bone density measurements. Her predicament is a reminder that exercise is only one part of the answer to perfect bones. Exercise must be balanced with proper nutrition designed for your particular body's needs.

As Mary Jane Mack, R.N., points out, "When bodies are deficient in the first place, exercise will be hard and people won't get to peak performance. They feel tired. People may drive themselves, but underneath they're still deficient in nutrients, which means they lack the nutritional foundation to fuel the process. Exercising alone cannot correct the deficiency, and may do more harm. One example is when people's heart electricity is low, and they drive themselves to exercise. If their main battery [their heart] is weak, then the whole system will weaken. After short or long term, their body can't handle it, and they wind up with more chronic problems . . . including stress fractures or more serious types of fractures, among other things."[18]

That's why Bruce West, D.C., puts people who need to rebuild their bones on concentrated nutritional protocols for thirty to sixty days before recommending they start exercising, and then insists they have a trainer. "They are in a real catch-22. Most are in relatively severe pain which makes them immobile, but they need to be active to recover. That's why they have to have a trainer. Almost anyone can develop a weight-bearing program—paraplegics, anybody. It may seem like a minor amount of weight, but even a tiny amount of weight will help."[19]

METABOLIC ACTIVITY

Physical (voluntary) activity speeds up metabolic (involuntary) activity, the rate at which the body breaks down and uses food. Therefore good digestive activity and absorption of foods is central to the good blood quality upon which bones depend. As Michael Dobbins, D.C., points out, "We are what we eat, based on what we metabolize."[20] In other words, to improve our nutritional state, we must not only eat well, but metabolize well. Metabolism can be understood in terms of digestive movement.

The materials in food become bone after being processed and absorbed in different parts of the digestive system. Although located inside the body, this system is actually a continuation of the outside of the body. Its mucous lining (mucosa) and cells are an extension of the skin. The digestive lining helps keep the outside out; if that protective lining breaks down, unwanted particles can get into the body. The digestive lining is not only the first line of absorption, it's also the first line of defense.

When digestion doesn't work properly, bones don't receive the deposits they need. The sometimes noisy and obvious symptoms of digestive problems can be a first indication that bone health is also declining. Such symptoms often include: bloating, belching, gas, diarrhea or constipation, stomach or intestinal pain, food allergies, rectal itching, and acne.

Digestive insufficiencies are also associated with certain diseases. According to the American Council on Collaborative Medicine, these diseases include: Addison's disease, asthma, celiac disease, dermatitis herpetiformis, diabetes mellitus, chronic hives and eczema, gallbladder disease, chronic autoimmune disorders, hepatitis, lupus erythematosus, myasthenia gravis, osteoporosis, pernicious anemia, psoriasis, rheumatoid arthritis, rosacea, Sjoegren's syndrome, thyrotoxicosis, hyper- and hypothyroidism, and vitiligo.[21]

Four main digestive areas carry out the activities that keep bones healthy: the mouth, the stomach, the small intestine, and the large intestine.

Mouth

The mouth serves as a reception room for materials destined for the bone bank. It is here that foods are received, registered, and begin their conversion into healthy bone bank deposits. Two events take place to initiate this modification process. The first is mechanical: the act of chewing. The second is the release of the enzyme ptyalin by the salivary, or parotid, glands.

Mixing food with ptyalin in the chewing process is the first line of defense within the digestive system; this secretion contains some immune cells (immunoglobulins) that begin to neutralize anything that could ultimately harm bones. Ptyalin also begins breaking down carbohydrates into a form that the stomach can receive (maltose and dextrin). Thus, lack of sufficient chewing or lack of sufficient ptyalin mixed with food renders it unavailable to the rest of the metabolic cycle and ultimately to the bones. But whether sufficiently chewed or not, once swallowed, food descends to the next digestive room, the stomach.

Stomach

In the second processing room, future bone bank deposits mix with gastric juices that contain various enzymes that break them down further. Sufficient hydrochloric acid (HCl) in the stomach is an absolute precondition for absorbing the nutrients that bones need. In fact, the calcium that bones require can only be absorbed in a sufficiently acidic stomach environment.

That's why it's self-defeating to take a calcium-based antacid and expect bones to benefit from the calcium content. Such antacids render the stomach too low in acid to complete its tasks. The body has to contend somehow with the unmetabolized calcium and often deposits it in the wrong places. That's one way calcium ends up in soft tissues. In artery walls it can cause atherosclerosis (hardening of the arteries). In the gallbladder it becomes gallstones. In the kidney, this calcium forms kidney stones. If deposited in the eardrum, it can harden the filmy eardrum and prevent it from vibrating, thus contributing to deafness.

Indeed, practitioner Mary Jane Mack, R.N., says the most common digestive problem that contributes to poor bone health is "lack of hydrochloric acid." That's why she evaluates all her clients to see whether they're able to absorb bone nutrients. If not, she adds Zypan (SP) or Betaine Hydrochloride (SP) to their protocols (see below). She says some people are unable to take either product because the mucosal lining of their stomach is so thin they can't handle ingesting this nutrition. In that case, she recommends Okra Pepsin E_3 (SP). Sometimes, depending on how much healing the stomach needs, she's had to "start people very slowly to get them absorbing nutrition before even starting to deliver the other nutrients they need." This circumstance, she points out, is most common in people whose "blood quality is very low, so low they can't even handle the nutrition. In turn, the most common causes of that are parasites or chemicals in the system that deplete the blood" (see chapter 11).[22]

Low levels of the mineral zinc are another factor when foods are not properly metabolized (see also chapters 6 and 7). This is especially likely when someone experiences many food cravings, often because the body craves the cofactors that help the stomach work. One of those cofactors is zinc. Zinc is needed for every bodily process because it is an essential component of all the bodily tissues that develop from the ectoderm—the outer layer of cells in a developing embryo. These tissues include all the skin structures, of which the entire gut is one, the nervous system, organs of special sense (nose, eyes, and ears), the pineal gland, and part of the pituitary and suprarenal glands.

Michael Dobbins, D.C., points to stomach ulcers as another disturbance that can contribute to poor bone health. "Stomach ulcers are bacterial invasions primarily due to lowered resistance due to vitamin deficiencies."[23] Since vitamins carry essential minerals into the bone bank, restoring healthy vitamin levels is a digestive key to perfect bones. Dr. Dobbins concludes, "Usually if you correct digestion in the stomach, you don't have to correct it below."

Small Intestine (Duodenum)

This is the third chamber for processing bone bank deposits. Foods are further digested here and then absorbed into the blood stream so they can be carried to the bone bank. For most nutrients, this is both their last and only chance to be absorbed.

To carry out its job, the small intestine receives some help. If dealing with carbohydrates, the pancreas sends assistance. In fact, the pancreas's role in bone health is being studied since it has been discovered that impaired glucose metabolism is associated with bone loss. For example, type two diabetics are known to have thick bones, but these bones still get fractures.

If fats are present in the small intestine, the gallbladder helps out by delivering bile (see chapter 8). If fats cannot be completely processed, there are several negative consequences for the bone bank. One is that the vitamins that fats are supposed to carry to bones cannot be absorbed, resulting in a deficiency of vitamins A, D, E, and K, despite adequate amounts in the diet. Another problem is that unmetabolized fats cannot provide courier service for minerals (see chapter 7).

Still another difficulty for bones can arise from incomplete protein breakdown, an activity carried out in this third digestive space. When proteins are incompletely digested, they cannot carry out their function of building the connective tissue mesh that receives bone bank deposits, thus weakening the connective tissue and, ultimately, the bones (see chapter 6).

Digestive processes in the intestine are greatly aided by friendly flora—intestinal bacteria. Without their help, digestion cannot be completed. That's a problem many people encounter as a result of taking antibiotics. These drugs destroy friendly intestinal flora along with disease-causing bacteria. Again, digestion remains incomplete, and bone-building nutrients cannot arrive at the bone bank. Also, without friendly intestinal bacteria, the stage is set for an overgrowth of undesirable microbes, such as yeast (candida), which embezzle bone nutrients and spend bones' riches on themselves (see chapter 11).

The relative health of the mucous membrane of the small intestine has everything to do with whether bones will get what they need. For example, if this membrane becomes damaged, it can leak. Usually, states Dr. Dobbins, this problem starts with an endocrine imbalance, which can result from a lack of the essential fatty acids that keep the mucous membrane healthy. That's why practitioners sometimes recommend Pituitrophin PMG (see chapter 9) for digestive system support: it is likely to help stimulate ulcers to heal.

The lining of the small intestine can, over time, become coated with a kind of internal sludge. This substance builds up in the same way that creosote does in fireplace chimneys. A tar-like substance coats the intestinal walls and prevents nutrients from being absorbed. This is especially likely for people with a high intake of refined carbohydrates and sugars. This unwelcome coating can be slowly removed by eating more dietary fiber.

Large Intestine

The last room in the digestive process acts as an exit station. The large intestine receives undigested remains of food from the small intestine. Rather than continuing to digest them, the large intestine moves them along (via peristalsis), removes water, and, with the help of friendly bacteria, further degrades them in preparation for elimination. Without this job taking place, undigested materials would back up in the system, contaminating and ultimately shutting down the metabolic processes that deliver bone bank nutrients.

Kidneys

The kidneys also contribute to healthy bones. They filter blood, remove other waste products, particularly sodium and potassium, and retain blood cells, proteins, and other necessary substances. Before eliminating what they have filtered, the kidneys provide one last service to the bone bank: they can selectively reabsorb calcium, magnesium, and potassium that had been destined for elimination, thus giving the bone bank a second chance to deposit them. The kidneys' ability to filter is dependent to a great extent on blood pressure, which is why it's so important to keep blood pressure in the normal range (around 120/80).

The kidneys also play a central role in maintaining proper pH balance. Without their constant vigilance in adjusting acid-base ratios, the nutrients that bones need could not be absorbed (see chapter 7). As Dr. Dobbins points out, "When there's a pH imbalance, it's always a kidney problem."[24]

ACTIVITIES DONE TO BONES

Both the voluntary movements of exercise and the passive movements of the metabolic cycle are affected by one other bodily activity: the movement of nerve impulses. If these impulses become blocked, the organs and muscles for which they were destined will never receive them. Without a free flow of nerve messages, the function of various organs and muscles will be inhibited. In turn, messages returning from these organs to the glands and areas of the brain that control them will not be delivered. The proper functioning of nerve impulses is the foundation of chiropractic practice. Since nutritional imbalances and deficiencies are often at the root of recurrent bone dislocations, or subluxations, many chiropractors include nutritional work as part of their practice.[25]

Because nerve impulses travel through the spine and near and around various other bones and joints, chiropractors adjust bones to align them so nerves that might be pinched are freed and become able to send their crucial messages to their destinations. When bones are out of alignment, they can cause difficulties with proper absorption. Whether misalignments are in the spine, wrists, shoulders, or ankles, it is important to bring bones back into alignment. However, a sudden adjustment can snap the bones of someone with severe osteoporosis. Therefore, make sure your body worker is aware of the state of your bone health, and refuse methods of adjustment that require sudden thrusts. There are other ways to produce good alignment that are gentle and equally effective. If your health care practitioner is a chiropractor, he or she will likely check your alignment and make necessary corrections.

In addition to chiropractic work, there is a gentle method of bodywork that provides direct stimulation to bones. Called Zero Balancing, and presented in the book of the same name authored by Fritz Smith, M.D., this method is both subtle and powerful. A trained practitioner can stimulate bones by applying slight pressure and movement to the muscles that attach to the bones.

Finally, since proper alignment is central to bone health, foot orthotics may be necessary to provide crucial support to the body's framework and organ systems. Certain health professionals are able to test for the need for orthotics.

RESTORING PROPER DIGESTIVE ACTIVITY

The following products are often recommended by practitioners as part of the protocols to help the digestive organs perform their metabolic functions.

Protocols are made from a combination of products as determined by your health practitioner. In the product descriptions below, "SP" designates Standard Process formulations, and "MH" designates those made by MediHerb. The sources for herbal information are *Principles and Practice of Phytotherapy: Modern Herbal Medicine*, by Simon Mills and Kerry Bone, and *MediHerb Innovative Herbal Solutions Product Catalog 2001*, unless otherwise noted. All products mentioned but not described here are detailed in other chapters (see index).

Products for Mouth Support

Paraplex (SP) provides nutritional support when low parotid (salivary gland) output is less critical than hormonal imbalances, especially in the pituitary, thyroid, pancreas, and adrenal glands.

Parotid PMG (SP) contains nutritional support for the parotid gland. It may be recommended to help rid the body of environmental toxins such as those from mercury amalgam dental fillings or from viruses that attack the parotid gland, such as mumps. It's also recommended in chemical poisoning, for people who've been on chemotherapy, or for those who were exposed to valley fever. Dr. Michael Dobbins reports that it's also excellent for people with silver amalgam fillings that are leaking, even if they don't get the tooth fixed.[26] Parotid PMG is also designed to support the relationship between the salivary glands (parotids) and the thyroid.

Vegetarian protocols for the mouth (parotid reflex) generally include Calsol, Choline, Spanish Black Radish, and Zymex II.

Products for Stomach Support

Betaine Hydrochloride (SP) is designed to make hydrochloric acid, which aids in the digestion of proteins and minerals, available to the stomach. Betaine is often recommended for people suffering from gas, indigestion, malassimilation, demineralization, and pernicious anemia.

Fucus Plus (North American Pharmacal) contains bladderwrack and larch, herbs that combine "to help normalize the sluggish metabolic rate and enhance weight loss."[27] It also supports intestinal and stomach lining.

Gastrex (SP) contains okra powder, discussed below, and bentonite (nutritional clay). It is often recommended to immediately relieve an overly acidic stomach. The clay's function is to draw toxins to itself for removal. Gastrex also contains *Tillandsia*, which lubricates, absorbs, and helps eliminate. Together, the combination helps put out the fire (inflammation), eliminate toxins, and provide a mucous membrane healing agent, okra pepsin.

Okra Pepsin E$_3$ (SP) provides nutritional support to help break down mucus when there's so much covering the intestinal wall that food can't be readily absorbed into the blood. Okra is sticky and adheres to the intestinal wall long enough to put the protein-digesting enzyme, pepsin, in contact with the protein-based mucus. It's especially helpful in colitis, diverticulitis, ulcers, malabsorption syndrome, and ileocecal valve problems.

Dr. Michael Dobbins adds that it "has the factors found in cabbage juice that have such healing powers. Therefore it has a role in addressing diarrhea, constipation, indigestion, intestinal flu, colitis, and gouty diathesis. It also contains vitamin E factors and other agents that support tissue repair."[28] He recommends taking it on an empty stomach so it can coat the stomach directly, without interference from food.[29]

Zinc-Liver Chelate (SP) provides the zinc necessary to activate the digestive processes. Because zinc feeds all the organs that arise from the ectoderm (listed previously in this chapter), it is useful for digestive insufficiencies, nervous system disorders, immune insufficiency, slow rates of healing, reduced sex drive, prostatic hypertrophy, loss of sense of smell and/or taste, chronic yeast infections, failing eyesight, hair loss, and gray hair. Zinc also needs to be present so vitamin D can work. White spots in the fingernails are one indication of zinc deficiency. Zinc always needs to be balanced with copper for optimum body functioning.

Zypan (SP) aids the stomach's digestive process by helping to normalize its acidity, which should be highly acid, at a pH of two or three. Zypan is therefore central to the absorption of calcium and iron. It also helps the stomach digest carbohydrates, fats, and proteins.

Vegetarian products for the stomach generally include Black Currant Seed Oil, Chlorophyll Complex, and Fen-Gre. Vegetarian protocols for the gut generally include Zymex II.

Products for Small Intestine Support

Betafood (SP, vegetarian) and **A-F Betafood** (SP) support the gallbladder and breakdown of oils (see chapter 8).

Cataplex GTF (SP) contains food factors that help increase insulin production in the pancreas and the cells' response to insulin. It is often recommended for nutritional support for low blood sugar (hypoglycemia), high blood sugar (hyperglycemia), or insulin production problems. It may also be used for its antiarteriosclerosis function, as research points to its help retarding the formation of arterial plaques of cholesterol and calcium that can adhere to the blood vessel walls.

Chezyn (SP) aids small intestine function and healing by providing zinc and copper, which help heal mucous membranes (see chapter 7).

DiGest Photosynergist (MH, vegetarian) is a liquid formulation of herbs specifically combined to promote digestion by strengthening and toning the whole upper digestive system. The combination acts to stimulate the appetite and increase digestive secretions, thus improving the breakdown and assimilation of food. It also helps settle digestive spasms and reduce flatulence. These actions mean food is less likely to remain undigested, thus reducing or even eliminating the toxic load on the body, which can be dangerous to connective tissue.

Gastro-Fiber (SP, vegetarian) contains phytonutrients from five different whole foods and botanicals. The phytonutrients function synergistically to help cleanse and lubricate the intestines, encourage regular elimination, promote pH balance through the gastrointestinal tract, and provide an optimal environment for the natural growth of friendly intestinal bacteria.

Vegetarian protocols for the small intestine generally include Linum B_6, Fen-Gre, and Lact-Enz. Vegetarian protocols for the pancreas generally include Inositol, Lact-Enz, Betafood, and Spanish Black Radish.

Products for Large Intestine Support

Spanish Black Radish (SP, vegetarian) is a large intestine detoxifier (see chapter 11).

Products for Kidney Support

A-C Carbamide (SP, vegetarian) contains a variety of nutritional factors that support the transfer of body fluids through cell walls. That process is called osmosis; it allows elements dissolved in liquid solution to pass through cell membranes. Osmosis enables nutritional elements to be used for cell metabolism or to carry out products of elimination. A-C Carbamide may be recommended for someone who is retaining water, has swollen extremities, has sweat gland symptoms, or has kidney and bladder symptoms, including the stimulation of nightmares. (See also chapter 9.)

Albaplex (SP) helps to support proper kidney function (see chapter 11).

Vegetarian protocols for the kidneys generally include A-C Carbamide, Spanish Black Radish, Zymex, and Organic Iodine.

Becoming physically active, supporting the digestive process, and freeing up nerve impulse transmissions through proper bone alignment can make all the difference in the quest for healthy bones. But there is one more factor to address. The bone bank must have protection from embezzlers, the subject of chapter 11.

ELEVEN

Strengthening Security Systems: Protecting Bones from Robbers, Embezzlers, and Leachers

WHEREVER THERE ARE RICHES, there are likely to be attempts to waylay them. The mineral treasures meant for bones are certainly no exception. Robbers, embezzlers, and leachers stand ready to remove hard-won bone bank deposits during any lapse in security. Thus, the final component of the Six-Point Plan for Healthy Bones addresses how to sustain sufficient protection to keep bone banks secure.

Bones have always needed protection. However, safeguarding them in the modern world is more important than ever before. Air pollution, for example, adversely impacts four to five billion people worldwide. Mary Jane Mack, R.N., explains the connection to bone health: "More people are deficient [in bone-building nutrients] today because of indoor and outdoor pollution. The houses are so well insulated, they don't breathe. The house has no filter system, so pollution builds up in the house. Many chemicals are used in cleaning, new products in houses, weed and feed chemicals around the houses, chemical lawns. These are all toxins that deplete the blood. People feel sick after they spray their yard, then they go to a resort to get better, but that place is sprayed with chemicals inside and out."

She continues, "And then there's radiation in the air from computers, cell phones, pagers. These emissions deplete the blood, the vitamins and iron, because the body can't handle it; it's like a foreign substance. These pollutants are at such levels today that the average person has a hard time keeping above it. If your body's a little unhealthy in the first place, you don't have a chance. Osteoporosis is the end result. The most common cause is the outdoor pollution. Women have achy bones; because their bones swell, they'll complain of joint or bone aches. I'm seeing it more in men now too."[1]

Sources suggest that "Americans are threatened daily by over 100,000 different synthetic chemicals. Shockingly, there are over one-half trillion pounds in the United States alone!"[2] And an estimated one thousand new chemicals are introduced every year, only a couple hundred of which have been tested for health effects. And of those that have been tested, few have been checked for health effects in children and developing infants.[3] This means the bone health of the new generation may already be severely impacted, long before they reach the officially recognized at-risk years for declining bone health.

In fact, the U.S. government is stepping up research on many of these chemicals because they may be "hormone disrupting," the signs of which are unnaturally early puberty for girls, lower sperm counts in men, increased rates of cancer, sterility, and developmental problems.[4]

It all adds up to the need for a strong, effective security system to protect bone bank deposits. Maintaining a security system that is truly effective requires some knowledge of the modus operandi of the various nefarious culprits. Knowing how they work provides solutions for preventing them from getting away with the bones' treasures. And, astonishing as it may seem, the most frequently encountered bone robber wears a friendly, familiar face: the food in the modern diet.

FOOD

Few people would consciously decide to give up long-term bone health by inviting known bone robbers to take up bodily residence. Yet that is exactly what happens on a daily basis when we consume many modern "foods." To comprehend the role of modern food-stuffs in damaging bones, step behind the scenes of contemporary food production and discover processes that could confound a rocket scientist.

The story begins with seeds (many now genetically altered) that are grown on depleted soil that is soaked with chemical fertilizers. This food is then sprayed with pesticides during its growth. (For an excellent and thorough treatment of this subject, see Jensen and Anderson's *Empty Harvest*.)

From there, reports Alan Gaby, M.D., modern food is "bleached, radiated, extracted with organic solvents, subjected to enormous temperatures and extremes of acidity or alkalinity and contaminated with thousands of chemicals designed to preserve, texturize, color, or otherwise modify the food so that it will look, feel, and taste like the real thing."[5]

The results of these processes are foods that look like foods, but act in the body like what nutritionist Bob LeRoy, R.D., labels "calcium antagonists." However they are labeled, the more processed food we consume, the more negative the ramifications for bone health.

Mary Jane Mack, R.N., explains that processed foods are electrically negative (levo-rotatory), while those that promote bone health (and overall health) are electrically positive (dextro-rotatory). Muscle-testing practitioners can actually test the electrical charge of a food the same way they can test the charge of a body reflex. "If an orange or an apple is really healthy, new, organic, it's more likely to test positive," Dr. Mack says.[6] In general, live, fresh, whole foods are positively charged, while processed, chemically preserved, highly sugared foods or old and stale ones are negatively charged.

Dr. Mack adds, "Positive foods spin to the right, and they build the body up at a cellular level; they give the person more energy and make the body healthier. Anything negatively charged pulls the health of the body down; it moves through the body slowly, therefore causing debris, which can even cause stones. Negatively charged food causes buildup in the liver and gallbladder: sludge. A lot of synthetic vitamins are negatively charged."[7]

Electrically negative foods force the human body to make dangerous substitutions in its structure. The body takes in and uses these counterfeit and imitation foods and chemicals in an attempt to compensate for the lack of natural elements. When natural elements are missing, the body is in a weakened state, allowing microbes to more easily embezzle and rob the remaining riches.

Such foods substitute chemicals for real mineral treasure and lower the effectiveness of the bone bank's security system, two reasons that nutritionist Bob LeRoy, R.D., defines negatively charged food as part of a "calcium-draining lifestyle." He says, "Evidence is mounting . . . that osteoporosis is not a disease of calcium deficiency, but rather the result of lifestyle choices that speed up calcium excretion from the bones. Consuming massive doses of calcium, whether through falsely-reassuring dairy products or mega-supplements, cannot be expected to counteract a 'calcium draining' lifestyle."[8]

He insists that we need to reduce, and in some cases avoid, the "calcium antagonists" over which we have control. These include: "above all others, animal protein and excess total protein; importantly, sedentary habits; and, to varying degrees, sodium chloride, smoking, vitamin D overdosing or sunlight deprivation, caffeine, steroids, alcoholism, aluminum, fluorides, refined sweeteners, and serious calcium/ magnesium or calcium/phosphorus dietary imbalances."[9]

Other experts concur. In fact, the National Institutes of Health issued a statement summarizing the present consensus: "Urinary loss accounts for approximately 50 percent [of calcium loss]. The typical American diet consists of high amounts of sodium and animal protein, both of which can significantly increase urinary calcium excretion."[10]

Food that was healthy to begin with, when undigested, can turn to poison in the body, attacking the very systems it was consumed to support.[11] This is how digestive problems contribute to a "calcium-draining" lifestyle. One factor that can lead to food remaining unassimilated is a pH imbalance. The more the pH balance is off, the more difficulty the body has healing. Undigested food actually putrefies and throws off pH balance with the result that food that should nourish instead literally attacks the body. Overeating contributes to making the body too alkaline, as does sleep deprivation.

Food allergies may also contribute to poor bone health. Since foods to which one is allergic are incompletely digested, they change bodily pH and reduce absorption of essential nutrients. To determine food intolerances, practitioners may recommend an elimination diet: removing a suspected food from the diet for a period of time and then adding it again to see whether it causes a reaction. Another method is to eliminate the foods one's blood type has difficulty tolerating. (See the lists in Peter D'Adamo's *Eat Right 4 Your Type*.)

While the scientific community has criticized Dr. D'Adamo's work for lack of sufficient research, clinical experience demonstrates that, for many people, not eating right for their type unbalances their hormonal systems, knocking their progesterone, estrogen, testosterone, and, especially, pancreatic hormone levels down significantly so they cannot build bone. In some cases, such inappropriate foods can knock the hormonal systems out of commission entirely.

Refined carbohydrates and sugar are high on the inventory of negatively charged foods and foods that have a profound negative effect on bone health. Because they contain few or no vitamins or minerals themselves, these foods, in order to be metabolized, use the riches meant for the bone bank. In other words, these foods rob the bone bank of its mineral deposits. Additionally, sugar actually causes the body to release calcium. As Alan Gaby, M.D., states, "Since 99% of the total-body calcium is in our bones, this increase in calcium excretion most likely reflects a leaching of calcium from bone."[12] Nutritionist Royal Lee, D.D.S., stated that glucose (the most common sugar we consume) blocks the assimilation of calcium.[13]

A recent study by researchers at the U.S. Department of Agriculture reported that "drinking lots of non-diet soft drinks can weaken your bones . . . the fructose sweetener in the [non-diet] drinks led to severe losses of bone-building phosphorous and calcium." This already bad situation is worsened fivefold in people whose magnesium intake is low.[14]

Bone-robbing sugar consumption has dramatically increased in recent decades. Sugar consumption was five pounds per person per year in 1930, and now it is two hundred pounds per person per year. One form of sugar that is particularly harmful to bones is corn syrup, which is added to breakfast cereals, fruit drinks, and a host of other foods. States Bruce West, D.C., "It is the only sugar that causes diabetes in test animals because it destroys the pancreas' insulin producing cells. It also blocks the assimilation of calcium in your body. And the end result can be osteoporosis and arthritis, two other epidemic diseases in this country."[15]

How drastically should we restrict our sugar consumption? Mary Jane Mack, R.N., answers that if sugar "is just one ingredient [of the meal], I don't worry about it. When someone is in a critical state of health and is severely depleted nutritionally, though, they have a hard time managing sugar. They don't realize until they get off it, how tired they were from trying to handle the sugar. Taking a lot of sugar daily depletes the nutrition in the body; it weakens their system and opens it for breakdown, including osteoporosis."[16] To give the body the nutrient it really needs when it signals a sugar craving, she recommends taking Inositol, one of the B vitamins (see below).

Alcohol is similar to sugar in its bone-robbing effect. People who drink excessively risk osteoporosis, partly due to the deficient diet that usually accompanies drinking, and partly due to the alcohol's toxicity. Alcohol dissolves and depletes the vitamin B complex, among other things. It is toxic to the liver, and it dissolves the crystalline mineral deposits held in the bone bank. As Michael Dobbins, D.C., points out, "Excessive alcohol ingestion destroys liver cells, which results in a massive tissue antibody response. In an otherwise healthy person this will normalize itself. The body produces histamine (in response to ingested toxins) which increases tissue permeability to help clean it out. Anti-histamines [either produced by the body or ingested] stop the histamine reaction. If the person stops ingesting alcohol soon enough, the liver will self-repair in a short time provided that the person is otherwise healthy."[17]

Caffeine is another bone leacher. It causes the body to excrete calcium at a rapid rate. Routinely ingesting a lot of caffeine, either in colas, coffee, or strong black teas, forces the bone bank into a deficit spending mode.

Smoking tobacco also has a direct negative effect on bones, although the reasons for this are not completely understood. The nicotine in tobacco is closely related chemically to the nutrient niacinamide. Inhaling tobacco causes nicotine to take up residence where the niacinamide belongs, especially in the nerves. Smoking nicotine is addictive in part because it throws the body deeper and deeper into a niacinamide deficit, which accounts for the frayed nerves of a smoker craving a cigarette. Part of smoking's negative effect on bones is presumed to be from toxins or chemicals in the smoke (such as the metal cadmium).

Does this mean that to keep our bone bank secure, we have to rigidly avoid all negatively charged foods and substances? No, says Michael Dobbins, D.C. He points out that even "Royal Lee said, in a well-fed individual, the body can deal with a little smoking and drinking. It's not the tobacco or alcohol [or sugar or caffeine] alone, it's the [combination of these toxins with] the debilitated state, and now the denatured food."[18]

There are two categories of foods that, by their very nature, are bone robbers and, therefore, should be ingested only in moderation. The first of these contains oxalates, as is found in spinach. Spinach is often recommended as a food high in iron. But iron competes with calcium, so spinach should be consumed separately from any calcium source, and then in moderation due to its oxylate content. The second group contains phytates, which are found in soy and the husks of various cereal grains. Both oxalates and phytates combine with calcium in the intestine and interfere with its absorption.

Modern meat has become a problem for bones also. Steers are fed estrogen to increase their weight, and when people eat the meat they consume that estrogen. This can contribute to estrogen dominance (see appendix III for list of symptoms), which lies at the root of many health problems, including bone loss. The solution for meat eaters is to consume only free-range meat.

The effect of genetically engineered foods on bones is still unknown. Although the research is not in yet, 90 percent of consumers polled state they would avoid such foods if given a choice. They are pressuring stores and grocery chains to remove genetically engineered ingredients from shelves. However, most consumers are unaware of the fact that chemical and pharmaceutical corporations like Monsanto have deliberately introduced genes from viruses, bacteria, and other

organisms into the food supply, ostensibly to make crops less susceptible to certain diseases or insects, and they have successfully avoided
providing this information on the labels.

Manufacturers have already removed genetically engineered
foods from products they sell in Europe, while in the United States,
according to the Grocery Manufacturers of America, as much as 70
percent of the processed food in a typical grocery store contains genetically engineered organisms.[19]

Mention should also be made of a class of food/drug/chemical
called a "nutraceutical." Like the word, which combines "nutrition"
with "pharmaceutical," these substances are part food and part
chemical—not (yet) classified as drugs—that deliver a concentrated
form of a presumed bioactive agent from a food, presented in a non-
food form. Sometimes called "designer foods" or "functional foods,"
these patentable products may be altered to the point that they are
no longer foods. These synthetic or manufactured imitations of food
chemicals have added substances with presumed health effects.
They isolate fragments of foods, overlooking the synergy of the
whole food. The industry founded the American Nutraceutical
Association to foster their goals. They represent the largest-growing
segment of the U.S. food industry, with sales estimates between $64
and $92 billion per year.[20]

SYNTHETIC CHEMICALS

Maureen Schaub, whose hormonal imbalances contributed to bone
loss, as described in chapter 9, learned that her occupation exposed
her to bone-robbing toxic chemicals. As a beautician, she was constantly breathing them in from hair dyes, perms, and other chemical
agents. Even though she had significant hormonal imbalances, her
body needed to deal with chemical poisoning as the first priority in

regaining her bone health. Because she is still constantly exposed to chemicals at work, Maureen continues to take a daily dose of Parotid PMG (SP), a product designed to clean chemical poisons from the body.

For Sophia Tampinelli, whose many layers of healing were described in chapter 5, dealing with chemical poisoning was also the first layer on the road back to bone health. However, she does not know the source of these toxins. What she does know is that she had an enlarged heart and a fallen or collapsed body due to chemical poisoning. Like Maureen, she took Parotid PMG. Although her practitioner also found hormonal imbalances, she was concerned that Sophia's heart was too weak to withstand the loss of fluids that she'd experience during her second layer of healing, sex hormone support. The Parotid PMG protocol would strengthen her heart enough to successfully pump out a massive release of fluids during her second layer of healing. Indeed, this proved to be true; Sophia lost twenty-four pounds of fluids in the first few months of her sex hormone protocol.

It is not surprising that Sophia was unaware of the source of her chemical poisoning. The average person in the United States is exposed to over a hundred thousand synthetic chemicals, including air and water pollution, pesticides, chemicals, synthetic drugs, synthetic vitamins in food additives, carpeting, paint, cosmetics, and more.

One important source of chemical poisoning is prescription drugs. Although they usually support health, drugs prescribed for an apparently unrelated symptom can rob bones directly or compromise the bone bank security system, leaving bones susceptible to being plundered. For example, as pointed out in chapter 9, keeping hormone factories in good production is central to bone health. But Dan Newell, C.N., explains that drugs can cause "a shift in endocrine compensation. For example, someone who has been hypothyroid may have developed such a chloride-sodium shift which has created such a pH imbalance that that's what you're fighting primarily . . . which the drugs can cause."[21]

One circumstance in which drugs promote bone loss is taking standard pharmaceuticals for thyroid problems and for estrogen replacement at the same time. Estrogen will block the effect of the thyroid medication, reports John Lee, M.D. However, natural progesterone enhances utilization of thyroid hormone.[22]

The class of drugs called antibiotics can promote bone burglaries indirectly. Dr. Dobbins explains that antibiotics suppress the immune system's signals to spring into action.[23] While the body's security system is dampened, antibiotics inadvertently make the bone bank accessible to burglars.

A partial list of other prescription drugs that have a bone-robbing effect can be found in chapter 3 under treatments that damage bones. The more such drugs are combined, the less anyone, even one's primary physician, can understand their effects. According to Bruce West, D.C., "if just three prescriptions are given, it is now considered a general fact that no doctor or pharmacist can understand the myriad of dangerous interactions between these drugs, your disease, and your body."[24]

METALS

Metals are a class of substances whose members can negatively impact bone deposits by displacing or replacing minerals that are vital to bones. They include aluminum, arsenic, barium, beryllium, bismuth, cadmium, cobalt, copper, iron, lead, manganese, strontium, and vanadium.

Aluminum is high on the list of such offenders. It accumulates in bones, reducing new bone bank deposits, speeding up bone bank withdrawals, and stimulating urinary excretion. Aluminum also interferes with the construction of the collagen net that receives deposits; thus, it participates in destroying the bank itself.[25] Avoid ingesting toxic aluminum by:

- Consuming juice or soft drinks from glass bottles, not cans or aluminum-lined cartons
- Consuming only aluminum-free antacids
- Using stainless steel or glass cooking utensils
- Filtering drinking and cooking water, or using bottled water from a reputable company
- Avoiding processed foods, as these often contain aluminum
- Refraining from using underarm deodorants that contain aluminum (usually as aluminum chloride or other aluminum salts)

Lead is also a bone-robbing culprit. Apparently it displaces calcium in the bone bank, thus increasing the rate of calcium withdrawal. Additionally, lead interferes with the hormone progesterone, which is necessary for regulating the bone bank. According to Susan Brown, Ph.D., "Unacceptably high levels of lead are found in our air, water, food and soils."[26] Indeed, people with chronic lead poisoning show evidence of osteoporosis. "We cannot rule out the possibility that a lifetime of low-level lead exposure is one of the factors contributing to the epidemic of osteoporosis in industrialized societies,"states Alan Gaby, M.D.[27]

Excessive exposure to cadmium, which is especially concentrated in cigarette smoke, contributes to a softening of the bones and resultant fractures.[28]

In sufficient concentrations, tin may reduce calcium content in bones. Tin also inhibits the production of hydrochloric acid in the stomach. Thus it prevents deposits from being processed and sent to the bone bank.[29] Tin is present in cans used to store food, toothpastes, some fungicides, insecticides, and stabilizers, in packaging materials, and in the atmosphere as an industrial pollutant.

Silver amalgam tooth fillings also contribute to osteoporosis because they can leak mercury. According to Megan Flaherty, "Mercury is a bioaccumulative neurotoxin linked to damage to the brain, kidneys and fetuses."[30] Donald Warren, D.D.S., states, "There always seems to be an increased plaque deposit around mercury amalgam restorations. The plaque toxin and the electro-galvanic current created by that restoration can accelerate bone loss adjacent to the filling."[31] Luckily, according to the *Price-Pottenger Foundation Newsletter*, "The fresh leaves of cilantro have been shown to mobilize mercury and other toxic metals from the central nervous system if large enough amounts are consumed daily. . . . Dried cilantro does not work."[32] Chewing cilantro with mercury-filled teeth, however, will pull the mercury from the filling, allowing it to be swallowed.

INFECTIONS

A nutritionally deficient body filled with synthetic chemicals and drugs is an environment weakened to the point of being unable to defend itself against disease-causing microorganisms. In turn, these living invaders wreak havoc on the mineral treasure intended for the bone bank. Whether bacterial, viral, parasitic, or yeast, each infectious agent interferes with the metabolic cycle of bone bank deposits and withdrawals in its own unique way. For example, bacteria such as staph (staphylococcus) or strep (streptococcus) not only eat bone, but also secrete toxins that harm bones.

Yeasts, such as monilia or candida, can suffocate the oxygen supply needed for bones' metabolic processes. Candida is especially relevant today because of the overuse of antibiotics. These kill off the normal flora in the intestines that are part of the intestinal tract's security system. Without these healthy bugs, yeast overgrows, crosses through the intestinal membrane, and spreads throughout the body. Systemically, it uses up bone nutrients, including precious oxygen. And yeast doesn't help digest food the way its friendly cousins, the intestinal bacteria, do; thus deposits intended for bone never reach the bank.

Viruses rob bones by entering into a cell and taking over the DNA that normally directs cell activities. Therefore viruses affect bones in a variety of ways, depending on the kind of virus and the kind of cells they take over. Viruses can seek out any kind of tissue, and are thus responsible for a wide range of symptoms and illnesses, including smallpox, chicken pox, measles, mumps, the common cold, rabies, epidemic breast cancer, prostate cancer, encephalitis, viral pneumonia, AIDS, and long-term chronic conditions such as fibromyalgia.

One way that viruses can affect bone health is by attacking connective tissue. This removes the collagen net where bone deposits are made, effectively getting rid of the bone bank itself. Viruses can also attack the nerve supply to bones or disrupt the circulation of blood to the bones. Nonetheless, "A virus in an environment that will allow it to replicate will do so, and will not in other environments," points out Dr. Dobbins.[33] Therefore, the key to avoiding such problems is to keep as healthy as possible so as not to provide an environment where viruses can reproduce.

Parasites are yet another form of bone robber. They consume the nutrition intended for bones, thus proliferating themselves while starving their host. Parasites are often found in people whose bone health is deteriorating. These uninvited guests can cause a host of symptoms, many of which may seem unrelated to an infestation, including abdominal pain or cramps, itchy skin, lack of appetite or increased hunger, autoimmune diseases, chronic fatigue, constipation, diarrhea, distention, fever, food allergies, gastritis, inflammatory bowel disease, low back pain, rash, weight loss, arthritis, colitis, flatulence, headaches, and vomiting, to name a few.

Fungi are vegetable cellular organisms that feed on organic matter such as bacteria and molds. Many fungi are not particularly pathogenic until they encounter a compromised, i.e., poorly nourished or unhealthy, host. For that reason, when fungi are present, health professionals suspect serious diseases. Some varieties of fungus that can cause primary infections occur in particular geographic regions, such as coccidioidomycoses in the southwestern United States, histoplasmosis in the eastern and midwestern United States, and paracoccidioidomycoses in South America. Because fungi feed on organic matter, they can eat the friendly bacteria needed in the gastrointestinal tract, leaving the digestive process incomplete. Fungi can also enter the system through decayed teeth, which are themselves a sign of compromised bone health.

The key to fighting off all these bone robbers is a healthy immune system. And, as Dr. Dobbins points out, "The fuel to run the immune system is calcium. The [immune] cells push out little ladders during phagocytosis; these are crystalline based and require calcium.

"The immune system is the only thing that can permanently destroy a virus. The immune system has to plug up the holes in the cell that allow those viral pieces through the cell wall and into the cell's DNA. . . . The immune system will plug up the hole in the cell wall with antibodies, which takes time. The viruses will *always* replicate when the environment allows it. The most important factor in this is calcium bicarbonate in the bloodstream and carbamide, which maintains the insulating values of the body fluids. In their deficiency, the nucleus and cytoplasm lose their opposite electrical charges, and the cell is dead when the charge is all gone."[34]

One new type of bone leacher is a thoroughly modern invention: nuclear power. The good news is that infection rates are lower near nuclear power plants, probably because nuclear energy kills microorganisms. The bad news, as stated earlier, is that such areas are intensely drying, using up the body's oils. What that means for bones, as described in chapter 8, is that there are too few carriers to transport minerals to the bone bank, and too few essential fatty acids to make sufficient hormones to regulate the bone bank. (Protocols for correcting these lapses in bone security are also in chapter 8.)

Before leaving the subject of robbers and embezzlers, a brief discussion of fluoride is warranted. As you may recall from chapter 3, fluoride has been put forth as a medical treatment for osteoporosis. Fluoride helps form bones and teeth, and it has been shown to increase bone mineral density test results. However, fluoride also renders these denser bones more brittle. Because it increases brittleness, fluoride can actually increase the likelihood of fractures. Bone mineral density studies do not measure the suppleness of bone, a factor that is as central to bone health as density.

For the body to utilize fluoride, plant life must first absorb the insoluble form from the soil. Chemical fluoride, which has not been rendered soluble through the action of plants, makes teeth softer, not harder, because calcium fluoride is not as hard a structure as calcium carbonate, the natural molecule in teeth. Nutritionist Royal Lee, D.D.S., pointed out that fluoride also inhibits and destroys vital enzymes essential for digestion and other metabolic functions. "In dilutions of one part in fifteen million, it's still poisonous enough to cut the activity of some enzymes as much as 50%." Without enzyme activity, he added, there is no life, no plant or animal that can live, so "anything that slows down enzyme activity is slowing down all life."[35] Fluoride molecules also clutch onto calcium and magnesium, essential for bone health, and eliminate them from the body.

John Yiamouyiannis, Ph.D., an internationally recognized authority on the biological effects of fluoride, reports that fluoride is a poison, slightly more poisonous than lead and slightly less poisonous than arsenic. He adds, "A spokesperson from Proctor and Gamble, the makers of Crest toothpaste, acknowledged that a family-sized tube of fluoride toothpaste 'theoretically, at least, contains enough fluoride to kill a small child.'" Fluoride is linked to weakened immune systems and the breakdown of proteins that form the structural framework (connective tissue) for skin, ligaments, muscles, bones, and teeth. Fluoridated water containing as little as one part per million has been shown to cause genetic damage—the same level that, in animal studies, has been shown to transform normal cells into cancer cells. Gastric cancer also has been associated with fluoride intake, and airborne fluoride has been linked to lung cancer.[36]

Last, a note about soft drinks. Soft drinks contain three to six teaspoons of sugar each and are loaded with phosphorus from phosphoric acid. Phosphorus combines readily with calcium. Therefore soft drinks can draw calcium out of storage in the bones and teeth, and their consumption can eventually lead to osteoporosis and decayed teeth.

REESTABLISHING EFFECTIVE SECURITY

Cleaning up chemical poisons in the body begins at their port of entry: the mouth. When health practitioners find a weak reflex in the hollow of a cheek, they often recommend Parotid PMG (SP) for chemical poisoning. Michael Smatt, D.C., who provided this care for Gloria Steinem in New York City, describes what's going on. "When functioning normally, the parotid hormones stimulate the production of saliva, which neutralizes toxins and digests bacteria and chemicals before they reach the rest of the digestive system."[37] The product Parotid PMG provides nutritional support to return these glands to peak functioning so they can clean up toxic chemicals (see chapter 10).[38]

After poisonous chemicals have been sufficiently eliminated from the body, practitioners often find the body in need of essential fatty acids, because the chemicals have dried up the body. If the reflex point located in the palm of each hand is weak, practitioners may recommend Linum B_6 (SP; see chapter 8).

When a particular liver reflex is weak, muscle-testing practitioners know that minerals and other substances backed up in the body need to be eliminated. When the liver can't eliminate these substances, the gastrointestinal tract and kidneys become stressed; these three systems (gut, liver, and kidneys) are buddies that cover for each other. If one can't get rid of a toxin, the other tries. When all three systems are overwhelmed, and the body is backed up with debris and wastes, it can lead to a condition called "incontinent bladder." If the liver is overstressed with too many chemicals assaulting the body, it knocks the bladder out of commission and fluid is retained. When excessive fluid is backed up, the legs and thighs may swell. The abdomen also may swell, and then fall, in some cases, nearly to the person's knees.

RESTORING A CLEAN ENVIRONMENT

To prevent bone robbers, embezzlers, and leachers, the body needs a regular supply of whole food nutrition to fuel the estimated six trillion chemical and electrical biological reactions that take place every second. The following products are often recommended. The best results are achieved when these products are combined with outdoor exercise in fresh air and sunlight. Ions of fresh oxygen, with their electrical energy, deliver what the red blood cells need to pump fresh oxygen to every cell and remove waste, including free radicals.

Mary Jane Mack, R.N., recommends positively charged juices (such as lemonade, cranberry, raspberry, pineapple, or orange) when the body is less toxic. Then she tests to see whether a client needs more protein, which is often the case if his or her blood quality was poor. She recommends clients choose foods that are electrically charged 80 percent positive and 20 percent negative because that combination "charges up the body electrically."[39] She tries to get the body balanced before making dietary changes because otherwise the person's appetite will be off balance. This is especially necessary for large people. When their blood quality is off, they fill up with water because the body's trying to protect itself.[40]

Regarding the body's cleansing process, Dr. Dobbins points out that when the correct product is given, the immune system starts to reset itself, and the result may be a histamine reaction. "By forty-eight to seventy-two hours, they'll have the symptoms of a cold. If you don't get the histamine reaction, it's not the right one. If they feel worse, that's the right one." Although it feels like their health is getting worse, this is actually a sign of getting better. To allow for that healing response, he recommends people, "*Always* work your way up, doing one pill the first day, two the second day, three the third day, et cetera, until you get to six."[41]

When someone is in the prodromal (initial) phase of an infection, Dr. Dobbins recommends using Organic Minerals (SP; see chapter 6). It supplies potassium to balance the part of the nervous system that controls involuntary functions (the autonomic system). It also provides calcium in its bicarbonate form, which, as Royal Lee pointed out, is the gatekeeper for the immune system.

For best results, most practitioners recommend chewing the products at least enough to break up the tablet's binding.

Protocols are made from a combination of products as determined by your health practitioner. In the product descriptions below, "SP" designates Standard Process formulations, and "MH" designates those made by MediHerb. The sources for herbal information are

Principles and Practice of Phytotherapy: Modern Herbal Medicine, by Simon Mills and Kerry Bone, and *MediHerb Innovative Herbal Solutions Product Catalog 2001*, unless otherwise noted. All products mentioned but not described here are detailed in other chapters (see index).

Whole Food Concentrates

Albaplex (SP) contains a combination of nutrients designed for kidney and liver support, especially for albuminuria (spilling of protein into the urine), which can indicate a pathological state of the kidneys, the onset of an infectious disease, or poisons in the body (either generated inside the body or from an outside source).

Allerplex (SP) provides upper respiratory nutritional support, especially when reactions to toxins result in troubled breathing. It includes nutritional factors that support the adrenal glands, liver, and lungs. It's often recommended for people who are food sensitive, are environmentally sensitive, or suffer from asthma and other lung problems except emphysema. Allerplex is often used in conjunction with Catalyn or another immune system support.

Antronex (SP) contains a natural antihistamine. It's often recommended when people develop asthma or allergies. It helps dry up the excess mucus that provides the medium in which infections can regrow. It also helps remove excess thyroxin (thyroid hormone) from the blood, so it may be suggested for people with a toxic thyroid.

Chlorella (Nature's Balance) is often used to detoxify the body of environmental pollutants from food, air, and water. Research has demonstrated that its cell wall attracts and binds with heavy-metal poisons such as lead, mercury, and cadmium and with hydrocarbon pesticides and insecticides such as DDT, PCB, and Kepone, thus enabling the body to eliminate them. Because chlorella is a toxic metal chelator, it can also bind with metals in the soil before it is put in products, causing the consumer to ingest the heavy metal along with the chelator; Nature's Balance chlorella does not have that problem. Chlorella is also a plant source of vitamin B_{12}, containing more B_{12} than beef liver. Nature's Balance has tested as being the most potent brand of chlorella available.[42]

Cholacol (SP) is for people who have severely depressed bile, such as someone who has undergone a cholecystectomy (removal of the gallbladder). It contains collinsonia root, a vascular astringent, which is often helpful for varicose veins.

Cholacol II (SP) supports toxic bowel clean-up. It helps when backed up toxins create a foul intestinal gas or a bad body odor. It helps clean people out fairly rapidly. However, there are often underlying liver and kidney problems that will need to be addressed afterward, Dr. Dobbins points out.

Choline (SP) acts as a physiological detergent. It is also a detoxifier that supports the liver. That's why it's often recommended for episodes of acute toxicity, such as sudden food poisoning. Choline makes the bile absorb the toxins so they can be eliminated.

Cilantro Extract (Nature's Balance) is a professional-grade, organically grown, and concentrated derivative of Chinese parsley (*Coriandrum sativum*). It is used to safely release mercury and other heavy metals from the body, including the brain. However, it is so effective at drawing out these substances that it must not be used until all metals have been removed from the mouth. A severe toxic reaction can result, which is why it is primarily available through health professionals who can supervise its use.

Collagen C (SP) draws fluids from the extremities to the bladder and kidneys. Practitioners may recommend Collagen C to return tissue fluid levels to normal.[43]

Congaplex (SP) provides nutritional support for people who keep getting strep infections. It contains a variety of nutrients to support the immune system, including calcium. Since it's water soluble, it's important to spread the dosages throughout the day so it doesn't just pass out of the body. Dr. Dobbins recommends taking it at the outset of feeling sick (the prodromal phase). He says at that point, "You've got about six hours to get this handled; otherwise you'll be sick ten to fourteen days." He adds that if you repeatedly get strep infections and have to take Congaplex, it's because you've only dealt with the acute phase; you need to rebuild your immune system with Immuplex (SP, see below).[44]

Cyruta Plus (SP) helps make the bodily environment more hostile to viruses. (See chapter 6.)

Echinacea-C (SP) is a source of herbs and other immune system boosters, including echinacea root powder, acerola powder, rose hip powder, and vacuum-dried buckwheat juice and seed. These are rich sources of calcium, copper, iron, manganese, phosphorus, potassium, B complex, and bioflavonoids that also help maintain connective tissue health.

Emphaplex (SP), states Dr. Dobbins, provides multiple nutritional factors for support "especially for people suffering from emphysema, or lung cancer."[45]

For-Til B$_{12}$ (SP) is often used in combination with Cal-Amo and Linum B$_6$ for nutritional support to deal with environmental toxins (see chapter 6).

Garlic (SP) protects against free radicals that damage body tissues. It also helps maintain normal cholesterol and triglyceride levels and a healthy flow of blood through the circulatory system. Each tablet is equivalent to one organically grown clove of whole garlic. Some practitioners use this form of garlic for its effect on the upper digestive tract.

Garlic (MH) is a liquid extract that is more effective for lower digestive and systemic applications, such as intestinal parasites, intestinal candida, and lowering cholesterol.

Immuplex (SP) provides nutrients—such as vitamin B_{12}, vitamin C, vitamin B_6, and folic acid—which support the immune system and the demands placed upon it by viral infections. It also provides nutritional factors that may be missing in people with long-standing immune deficiencies and autoimmune conditions.[46] Immuplex can be used concurrently with Congaplex (see above). It is usually taken for three months, but in difficult cases, such as fibromyalgia, Dr. Dobbins says, "A long-term chronic viral infection may need Immuplex for six months to a year or so."[47]

Inositol (SP) is part of the B complex of vitamins and is especially helpful for dealing with sugar cravings. It also supports the breakdown of fats.

Parotid PMG (SP) provides nutritional support for chemical poisoning. It's the product that both Maureen Schaub and Sophia Tampinelli took to heal their first layer in regaining their bone health. Dr. Dobbins reports giving Parotid PMG to one patient who "was allergic to everything. She had such a severe reaction she was absolutely laid up. She actually had to start with one-sixth of one Parotid a day." He points out that, in this case, "The worse the reaction, the better the result." He emphasized how important it is to start slowly. "If you've identified the right product to help them clean out, they'll have a reaction. That gives the patient a better understanding of what's going on, and then you can lower the dose to slow down the pace of the detoxification process."[48]

Spanish Black Radish (SP, vegetarian) is a colon-detoxifying herb, especially useful in quickly eliminating toxins such as those produced by the die-off of *Candida albicans* (yeast infections). It also supports the free action of the intestinal valves, the doors between the rooms of the gastrointestinal tract, so they can open easily and allow toxins to pass, and then close, so waste materials don't back flush and retoxify the system. (See also chapter 10.)

Dr. Dobbins adds, "Spanish Black Radish was developed to support people with colon cancer. It is for toxic bowel conditions. It's antiparasitic, and it's also good for liver congestion, diarrhea, virus, and constipation. It's high in sulforaphane, which grabs cancer cells. The person may need Cholacol II also."[49]

Thymex (SP) is often recommended as nutritional support for people who keep getting staph infections.

Zymex (SP) is recommended as nutritional support for toxic bowel problems, such as lower bowel gas, diarrhea, and constipation, and for intestinal overgrowth of yeast. Zymex contributes to making an acidic environment in which yeast cannot survive. It also contains enzymes that break down the yeast.[50] Zymex is frequently combined with Spanish Black Radish, Cal-Amo, and Lact-Enz, which contain healthy bacteria and enzymes that act as scavengers to clean up bodily pollution.

Zymex II (SP), not to be confused with Zymex, is recommended when parasites are a problem. It can also be used to prevent parasites when traveling to foreign countries. Because it contains factors that help digest protein, when taken on an empty stomach it digests the protein coating around the parasites.

Herbal Products for Liver Support

Dandelion Root (MH) is a liquid extract that supports healthy liver and gallbladder function by supporting bile production to digest fats, and by assisting the liver in filtering and neutralizing accumulated toxins. It also encourages natural function among the body's major organs of elimination. For those reasons, it is included in Colax tablets (MH), Livton Complex tablets (MH), and DiGest Phytosynergist liquid (MH).

Globe Artichoke (MH) supports healthy liver and gallbladder function. It is also included in Livton Complex tablets.

LivCo (MH) contains rosemary, which supports liver function. Rosemary can also be found in Bacopa Complex (MH) and Vitanox (MH, see chapter 6).

Livton Complex (MH, see chapter 8) contains both fringe tree and greater celandine, which support the liver.

Milk Thistle (MH) is a liquid extract that supports healthy liver function, encourages healthy protein synthesis, and promotes normal responses to environmental stresses. It also enhances healthy bowel function and provides antioxidant protection.

Schisandra Fruit (MH) is a liquid extract that helps cleanse the liver. In addition, it supports lung and adrenal gland function, stimulates the nervous system, enhances memory and mental clarity, supports and maintains cellular health, and supports lung and adrenal gland function.

Herbal Products for Stress Reduction

Eleuthero (Siberian Ginseng) (MH) is a liquid extract that enhances the body's natural ability to adapt to temporary stress. It also supports physical and mental endurance, promotes vitality, restores and enhances immune system function, and acts as a general tonic.

Hops (MH) is a liquid extract used to ease the effects of everyday stress and tension. It encourages relaxation, promotes healthy sleep patterns, and promotes appetite and healthy digestion.

Kava Kava (MH) is used to counteract states of anxiety. It works to ease the effects of temporary stress and to promote relaxation and sleep, during which times bones are built. It also promotes relaxation in both smooth and skeletal muscle tissue, thus reducing the body's demand for calcium, which muscles and skeletal tissue require to remain contracted. It is available in a liquid extract or tablet form. Because it is a relaxant, kava kava should not be taken at dosages greater than those recommended by the manufacturer or your practitioner. Also, you should get to know its effect on your body and take heed when considering driving a car or operating heavy machinery.

Skullcap (MH) is a liquid extract used to support the nervous system. It promotes relaxation and encourages sleep, and relaxes and soothes temporary tension associated with the menstrual cycle.

St. John's Wort (MH) is a liquid extract. Its popular reputation is due to its specific use for depression. However, it also demonstrates strong antiviral properties. Its phytochemicals support the body's natural ability to cope with the changes of everyday life and provide a tonic for the nervous system. St. John's wort helps ease the effects of occasional stress and promotes optimal immune response to environmental stresses.

Valerian (MH) supports bones by reducing the nervous system stress that contributes to a bone-leaching environment. It supports the nervous system, promotes relaxation, encourages sleep, and eases the effects of temporary or occasional stress.

Valerian Complex (MH) is a tablet that contains valerian, passionflower, and *Zizyphus spinosa*, a combination that works synergistically to help support the nervous system, promote relaxation, encourage sleep, and ease occasional stress.

Herbal Products for Inflammation Reduction

Andrographis Complex (MH) is a tablet that blends andrographis, echinacea root, and holy basil. Together they enhance immune system function, support healthy respiratory system function, encourage adaptive responses to occasional stress, and promote healthy liver function.

Boswellia Complex (MH) is a tablet that contains boswellia, celery seed, ginger, and turmeric. Together they act synergistically to support the kidney's normal function of clearing acidic waste products. It also helps maintain and support healthy joints, promotes the body's normal resistance function and healthy circulation, supports a healthy response to environmental stresses, and provides antioxidant protection.

Bupleurum (MH) is a liquid extract that promotes healthy liver function, stimulates protein synthesis, and promotes the body's normal resistance function.

Chamomile (MH) is a liquid extract that helps reduce gas buildup in the intestines, encourages relaxation, and supports a healthy nervous system response. It also supports healthy digestion and appetite and stimulates the body's normal tissue restoration functions.

Echinacea Premium (MH) tablets combine two types of the echinacea plant with calcium to enhance immune system function, including normal interferon production. (Interferon is a protein that certain body cells produce; it nonspecifically inhibits infection by a wide range of viruses.[51]) It also supports healthy white blood cells and encourages healthy upper respiratory tissue.

Ginger (MH) is a liquid extract that helps promote the body's normal resistance and supports a healthy response to environmental stresses. It also eases the effects of occasional upset stomach, promotes healthy circulation, cleanses the colon, and promotes healthy digestion. It has been used to support and maintain the body's normal temperature as well as to support healthy joints.

Saligesic (MH) contains white willow bark, often called nature's aspirin, which has been used for centuries to relieve pain and to lower fevers in conditions such as sore muscles, chills, rheumatism, or any inflammatory condition. It works against the prostaglandins in the body that produce inflammation. Unlike aspirin, it does not cause bleeding or gastrointestinal discomfort.

Turmeric (MH) is a liquid extract that provides antioxidant protection, supports healthy liver function and bile secretion, supports and enhances the proper breakdown of dietary fats, promotes normal platelet function and circulation, supports and maintains cellular health, promotes the body's normal, protective response to environmental stresses, and maintains and supports healthy joints.

Products for Maintaining Healthy Blood Sugar Levels

ARA6 (North American Pharmacal, vegetarian) is a powder containing larch, which is used to enhance immune function. It also acts to increase friendly bacteria.[52]

Gymnema (MH) can help suppress normal cravings for sugar. It also helps maintain healthy blood sugar levels when combined with a balanced diet, and it helps maintain normal cholesterol levels.

SP Cleanse (SP, vegetarian) is a combination of over twenty different whole foods and botanicals that have detoxifying properties. It helps the body eliminate toxins that originate in the environment. It also helps eliminate metabolic toxins that develop internally, such as when undigested food turns to poison. By supporting the body's internal waste-removal systems, it encourages healthy kidney function, helps purify the blood, supports lymphatic system function, promotes efficient gastrointestinal elimination, and maintains healthy liver detoxification functions.

Products for Cleansing Blood, Improving Lymphatic Circulation, Boosting Immunity, and Helping Clear Chronic Skin Conditions[53]

Burdock Root (MH) supports healthy blood, liver, and gallbladder function; encourages the organs of elimination to function optimally; boosts the immune system; and helps keep the skin healthy.

Calendula Flower (MH) encourages healthy menstrual cycles, promotes oral health, helps maintain healthy skin, and supports lymphatic system functioning.

Fresh Cleavers (MH) supports normal flushing of toxins, promotes healthy skin, and supports lymphatic functioning.

Goldenseal (MH) assists in maintaining healthy breathing passages, helps maintain healthy mucous membranes, supports the normal production and flow of bile, helps cleanse the gastrointestinal tract, and helps support the body's response to environmental stress.

Nettle Leaf (MH) supports the body's organs of elimination and functions of resistance (see chapter 6).

Red Clover Flower (MH) encourages the healthy function of the organs of elimination, promotes healthy skin, and helps maintain healthy blood.

Uva Ursi (MH) encourages healthy urinary tract function and tones and supports the genitourinary tract. It is often used to prevent or treat urinary tract infections.

Products for Other Conditions

To support the body with staph or strep, practioners may combine: Echinacea-C, Spanish Black Radish, Fen-Gre, Cal-Amo, and Lact-Enz.

To support the body in the presence of yeast, practitioners may combine: Zymex, Spanish Black Radish, Cal-Amo, and Lact-Enz.

To support the body in the presence of viruses, practitioners may combine: St John's wort, ARA6, Fen-Gre, Lact-Enz, Cal-Amo, and Calsol.

To support the body in the presence of parasites, practitioners may suggest: Zymex II.

To support the body in the presence of environmental toxins, practitioners may combine: Parotid PMG, Calsol, Choline, Spanish Black Radish, and Zymex.

To support the body exposed to environmental radiation or allergens, practitioners may combine: Linum B_6, Cal-Amo, and Spanish Black Radish.

The first five points of the Six-Point Plan for Healthy Bones explained how the bone bank develops and operates. Strengthening the security systems was Point Six. Part three will relate these points to the actions that produce success.

Kennet   Kennet

PART THREE

The Road to Perfect Bones

TWELVE

Proceeding

SINCE YOU'RE PROBABLY OVER TWENTY years old, you won't be able to build your peak bone mass. However, it's not too late for you to do something effective about assessing your bone bank status and making additional deposits if necessary. Nor is it too late to bring your account into proper balance so that your withdrawals don't exceed your deposits.

You can secure your future physical health the same way that you assure your future financial health: by investing in it. Finding out that you may be developing osteoporosis can turn out, like it did for me, to be a blessing in disguise. In taking the steps to turn it around, you learn how to rebuild various body systems and how to maintain your health. You not only improve your present health, but also invest in your future well-being.

Dan Newell, C.N., points out that "menopause is a great time to reevaluate what the last fifty years of your life have been. It's a great time to not just address symptoms, but bring the body back into balance."[1]

Jennie deMaria is preparing to do just that. Now forty-seven, she is entering her midlife phase. She has always eaten a good diet based on whole foods, and, up until now, she's been in excellent health. She has two healthy children and has stayed active as an avid hiker and gardener. In the last ten years, though, she's become more sedentary, in part because of working in an office. Now she fears the recent onset of symptoms is the beginning of osteoporosis, and she doesn't want that to happen.

She said, "After reading *Perfect Bones*, I recognized some of the characteristics of withdrawals from my bone bank, beginning thirteen years ago with broken teeth and a dark spot on my cheek. I do have the genetic predisposition: northern European, fair skinned. I'm part Italian and part German."

Some of Jennie's symptoms include: "A feeling of anxiety and feeling volatile, like anything could happen, and it wouldn't be anything good. I feel not only physically fragile, but emotionally fragile as well. I do have very brittle nails, toenails more than fingernails, for some odd reason." She has had a couple of night sweats, and her periods have changed from normal and regular to long (seven days instead of four) and frequent (two a month). They are now accompanied by headaches: "I get a premenstrual headache that no aspirin or ibuprofen can take away. It starts up to five days before the onset of my period and lasts the duration of my period. It doesn't happen any other time."

Her hair is now turning gray rapidly, and she's noticed that, "my lower back is always snapping in the morning. It's stiff and uncomfortable; it makes noise. When I stand up straighter, I hear it snap. It lessens as the day wears on, but then I might get it again in the evening. I have a condition called 'otosclerosis' [progressive deafness due to the formation of spongy bone around the stapes bone in the ear]. The stapes bone in my ear has grown too large to do its job of vibrating on the drum, so I have some hearing loss in one ear. I guess the nerve is damaged." (Since the body robs calcium from any bone to keep up blood levels, this ear condition may have resulted from calcium being borrowed from the stapes bone. If so, and if the nerve is not permanently damaged, it's possible she could regain this hearing loss as she balances her bone bank account.)

Jennie has also noted increasing heart palpitations. "I have a specific situation in my heart: mitral valve prolapse. I originally was diagnosed with a murmur when I was getting a physical to go to college. Later when I went for checkups when I was pregnant, a doctor diagnosed it as mitral valve prolapse [this condition is sometimes associated with magnesium deficiency], so I have to take massive antibiotics when I have dental work done, but that's a problem for me because I automatically get a yeast infection. I've probably had ten yeast infections in the last five years."

Jennie concludes, "I also feel like my strength in my bones in my arms and my stamina has diminished. I'm not as strong now as I was in my mid-thirties.

"I know that I need to supplement my calcium intake but haven't been able to figure out what form it should be in and what minerals it should be taken in combination with so it doesn't just pass through my body and do me harm. *Perfect Bones* has given me insight, and I now think there might be levels I need to take for different parts of my body to trigger natural body responses that help my bones. I want to know what my body specifically needs. I don't trust generic, over-the-counter dosages and one-size-fits-all drugs."

After reading *Perfect Bones,* Jennie wanted to be tested. Muscle testing revealed that two of the six points needed to be addressed right away: Point Four, balancing her hormonal system (specifically the adrenals and the pituitary), and Point Two, providing certain minerals and the helping vitamins to carry them into her bones.

After these discoveries, Jennie remarked that she was "in awe at the process of being tested. It reminds me of witnessing aikido masters because it's similar to the remarkable things they do with the flow of energy, such as a small person overpowering a large one. I'm amazed at how sensitive the tester is to me. There's something I don't really understand that's at work here. I felt for myself how my testing arm went weak in problem areas. It's heartening to know that people can tune into the body's mysterious circuitry like this and know how to work with it.

"I feel relieved that the problems in my body have been pin-pointed. I'm eager to try the protocols and experience the effect they'll have on me."

If, like Jennie, you too want to be tested, where do you locate a qual-ified practitioner?

THIRTEEN

Practitioners

HEALTH PRACTITIONERS who are competent to assess your unique nutritional needs and make recommendations can be found in a variety of professional ranks: physicians, nurses, chiropractors, dentists, naturopaths, nutritional consultants, dieticians, and, for animals, veterinarians.

Most clinical nutrition practitioners initially learn through personal experience and then decide to undertake training. Mary Jane Mack, R.N., for example, learned about nutritional products through her horses' veterinarian. When her sick horses got better in three months, she decided to attend a seminar, where the body was presented with "so much sense to me, with such easy solutions. I'd worked in labor, in delivery, surgical recovery, intensive care. By the end of the day, I knew that's what I was going to do." She began studying and attending seminars, and gradually the word spread. She never advertised, she said. "The more I learned, the more people appeared. It was word of mouth. They came and brought their families."[1]

Health care professionals in this field can be located in a variety of ways. Some practitioners are on the Internet. You can also contact Standard Process: visit their website at www.standardprocess.com, call 800-558-8740, or email info@standardprocess.com. Ask for a good,

active, well-trained practitioner in your area. If the recommended
practitioner is not taking new clients, ask them for a referral.

Many of these practitioners are chiropractors. Why have so many
chiropractors recently turned to nutrition? Michael Dobbins, D.C., a
former chiropractic college professor who now trains professionals in
clinical nutrition, has an idea about that. "At the turn of the century
the average diet was pretty good, so chiropractors did adjustments
and people got well. But now we're not feeding cells, and correcting a
nerve impulse problem won't do it."[2]

Get several names before selecting the right match. Since you're
going to be working with this person over time, you'll need to develop
a good, trusting, working relationship. Therefore, if you're the kind of
person who wants a scientifically oriented practitioner, you might
choose someone who can recite chapter and verse of a given metabolic
process's chemical pathways. Or you might choose a practitioner who
listens well and relates to you, understands your difficulties, and helps
you trust their recommendations. Some effective clinicians have the
bedside manner of a bull in a china shop; others have a gentler manner. The key is to find a practitioner who can help you restore your
bone health.

To evaluate the clinical nutrition practitioners on your list, consider the following:

- What training do they have?
- Do they attend workshops and keep up to date?
- Do they have previous experience?
- How long have they been practicing?
- How many people with osteoporosis have they helped?
- Are they improving your health or just pushing products?

Keep in mind that practitioners in one area of the country may have a
different emphasis from those in another area owing to different

dietary habits of the local population, regional soil and water conditions, and the availability of various foods.

Next consider how the person works. Practitioners structure their appointments and fees in a variety of ways. On one end of the spectrum are those who have you write down your symptoms prior to the appointment, read them off at the start of the session, then test you and design your protocol in just a few minutes. Their fees are likely to be lower because they are seeing large numbers of people per hour. The advantage is that it doesn't cost you much, you have an effective protocol, and, if you do what they suggest, you're likely to see good results.

In the middle range of the spectrum are practitioners who take a bit more time, perhaps a half hour, during which they assess you and listen to and address some of your concerns.

At the other end of the spectrum are clinicians who charge an hourly fee. They often integrate testing and designing your protocol with other kinds of healing work such as various forms of bodywork or counseling. This allows for the greatest individual attention, and, because it requires the most time with the practitioner, may come with the highest hourly fee.

Each type of practice has its strong points. What's important is for you to be clearly informed about your protocols and reassessments. It's no good getting a low rate on the testing fee if you don't have sufficient support from your practitioner to follow through. It's too easy to misread your own bodily changes as meaning something negative about the healing process. Your health care professional can keep you from becoming disheartened or quitting, reminding you that your goal is within reach.

Insurance coverage depends on the insurance carrier, the state in which your practitioner works, your practitioner's professional degree, and whether or not your practitioner accepts insurance payments. As of this writing, some insurance carriers cover nutritional counseling office visits but not the products, though a few with an eye to long-term savings are considering covering products.

Once you've decided on a practitioner, it will be time to learn which protocols are right for you.

FOURTEEN

Protocols and Products

ONCE YOU LAUNCH YOUR QUEST for perfect bones, you will be confronted by the vast array of nutritional products on the market today. Since sorting them out could take a lifetime, a better option is to work with an experienced health practitioner.

One of the first things you'll discover is that most practitioners recommend real herbs and whole food concentrates, products that truly support healing. If you're like I was, you may learn the truth of this the hard way. Initially I thought the difference between synthetic chemical isolates and whole food concentrates was marginal and didn't matter. I had taken whole food concentrates to restore my bones because that's what my practitioner recommended.

In the grocery store one day, I thought I'd pick up some vitamin C. I had enough sophistication to know that if the label didn't specifically say "no lactose," the product probably used lactose as filler and a tableting agent. (I am lactose intolerant.) I found a lactose-free product and purchased a generous-sized bottle. I took it as directed for several months, during which time my alignment wouldn't hold (a signal of weak adrenals or weak connective tissue). I could not figure it out. Finally my local health practitioner found the culprit: the "vitamin C" product actually contained only ascorbic acid, which is one small part of the whole vitamin C complex. This chemical isolate can actually be harmful in higher doses. I hadn't known the difference then, but my body certainly did. I reverted to whole food concentrates immediately and began to heal again.

A second experience—this time with a synthetic vitamin B complex—convinced me. I'd begun taking it to support my heart health, but a few weeks after starting to take it, I felt worse, weaker, like my heart was working even harder. At a professional seminar I had an acoustic electrocardiogram (the same thing as an EKG, except it uses sound to translate heart patterns onto graph paper). When tested with my synthetic vitamin B product, the heart graph flattened. The synthetic product was depressing all my heart functions.

Synthesized chemicals that imitate part of a whole food simply do not carry that food's healing power. Whole food concentrated to clinical potency heals wholly. That's why so many health practitioners who prefer true whole food concentrates use Standard Process products, and many use them exclusively. That's also why some scientific research projects that have studied nutrition's contributions to healing have had such mixed results. Many of the experiments used synthetic chemical isolates instead of whole food concentrates.

One way to ascertain whether the product you're considering is whole or synthetic is to read the label. You will recognize many names of foods and herbs, such as beets or tillandsia, but will not know the names of inorganic compounds, such as those that begin with *hydroxy-* or *tri-*. Also, if the product carries a patent number, it has been chemically altered, which is what makes it eligible to be patented. Whole foods cannot be patented. Again, your practitioner's expertise will guide you.

Osteoporosis, as we have seen, is a symptom, not a cause. Since each person's body is different, each plan for achieving perfect bones is unique. The trained practitioner tests to determine which problems to address and in what order. The body and its innate wisdom, with the assistance of a health professional, will guide you to healthy bones.

Yet, if you were to be tested by several practitioners, you might find yourself confused because they recommend different products. This variety is an indication, not of incompetence, but of the uniqueness of each practitioner's approach. The goal of perfect bone health can be approached from a variety of directions. Each practitioner may address the same general weaknesses with a particular emphasis, given their knowledge of various products, your state of health, and your priorities. As Dr. Dobbins puts it, "To choose a product, there's so much good stuff in everything. That's why we appear to have conflicting protocols . . . but when you give good nutrition, it feeds the system and they get well."[1]

Though each person is unique, Royal Lee, D.D.S., recommended a general protocol for people with osteoporosis that included ionizable calcium, raw bone enzyme protein factors, sex hormone precursors, prothrombin factor, potassium and trace mineral source, and calcium diffuser.[2] Other practitioners recommend different combinations based on what they find after assessing the individual. Combinations may include the following products: Cyro-Yeast, Calcium Lactate, Calcifood or Biost, Chlorophyll Complex, Organic Minerals, and Cataplex F.

If someone were to take one single product for improving their bone health, many practitioners would recommend e-Poise (SP). It builds blood, which in turn builds bone. E-poise was originally designed from recommendations by George Goodheart, D.C., who founded the healing system of Applied Kinesiology. E-Poise contains a multitude of nutrients that the body needs, including iron, vitamins, enzymes, herbs, and essential fatty acids. The combination of nutrients in e-Poise supports many of the points of the Six-Point Plan for Healthy Bones, including good blood quality and overall endocrine balance and support. E-Poise can provide what bones need if taken for a longer period of time, perhaps daily like a multivitamin. That's why e-Poise is likely to be recommended for young people looking for a good preventive product while they are still in relatively good health. As Dr. Michael Dobbins emphasizes, "There's benefit in a small amount long-term for maintenance also."[3] Other products and protocols are designed, for the most part, to support rebuilding certain organs or systems for a shorter period, often three months.

Mary Jane Mack, R.N., notices, "Most people on whom I pick up osteoporosis have been depleted in their blood for a long time, so they need e-Poise [included in their protocol]. That's the important preventative because it builds the blood and supports the bones. Without vitamins and iron, the bones become weak and can swell. That's what causes pain and makes a lot of people worry about their bones. Pain is their presenting complaint. Some people complain of achy joints, adjustments that don't hold . . . underneath they're deficient in vitamins and iron."[4]

Many people's health is too far out of balance or they don't have enough time to use e-Poise alone. To address the problem of poor blood quality and poor bone health from all angles, practitioners are likely to combine from the following products (all Standard Process) to design an effective protocol: Calcifood Wafers, e-Poise, Chlorophyll Complex Perle, Cataplex F Perle, Utrophin (female) or Prost-X (male), Mammary (female), Ovex (female) or Orchex (male), and Zypan, to aid digestion and absorption.[5]

Mack, who has used such a protocol with some of her clients, comments: "Using this protocol for osteoporosis, people are doing even better [than before it was devised]. People turn around faster; they notice a difference sooner. In twelve weeks you see big differences. It depends on what their state of health is. If you have to clean up deficiencies in the body first, it could take six months to a year. For example, things will go more slowly if you need to clean up chemicals or other things like bacteria that are weakening the system."[6]

If the person has or is prone to gout, practitioners take a different approach, and may recommend combinations that include Cataplex F Perles, Min-Tran, Chlorophyll Complex, and Zypan.

However, if someone needs more e-Poise a day, they might receive a protocol with a different underlying strategy, such as: Lact-Enz, e-Poise, Organic Iodine, Min-Tran, A-C Carbamide, Betafood, Zypan, and Chlorophyll complex. This type of protocol is designed to help the cells eliminate toxins and take in nutrition.[7]

Bruce West, D.C., whose newsletter *Health Alert* reaches thousands of subscribers, brings together a protocol to promote bone health that combines: Biost, Cal-Ma Plus, and Calcifood Wafers or Bio-Dent. If the person has involvement in the mandible (jawbone), teeth, or other bones of the face, Biodent is recommended in place of Calcifood Wafers. For vegetarians, Dr. West would likely include: Calcium Lactate and Chlorophyll Complex.

Dr. West emphasizes, "Each patient is different. The above are cookbook recipes only." He adds that he uses Standard Process products in part because "the way they design their products, they stimulate and normalize hormones."[8]

Dr. Michael Dobbins says that if he were to use just one product, he would choose Ferrofood (SP). "Ferrofood is the finest blood-building product on the market. Ferrous lactate doesn't constipate; it's far more assimilable. The body doesn't eliminate what it needs. Ferrofood contains bone meal, and nutritional support for the duodenum, spleen, adrenals, stomach, and liver."[9]

Nutritionist Royal Lee, D.D.S., states that bone pain is often due to a lack of raw food vitamins and amino acids, particularly lysine and tryptophan, that are affected by heat such as pasteurization, cooking, and autoclaving.[10] His recommendations often included: Catalyn or Cyrofood, Biost, Protefood, and Prost-X.

Your practitioner will help you decide what your body needs. During your appointment, communicate your priorities clearly. Is your current goal, for example, to chase down a symptom that's been bothering you, or are you interested in general health improvement, or are you looking for a personalized program for improving your bone health? Many practitioners will ask you to bring in a list of what you want.

Once you have your practitioner's recommendations, it's time to decide what products to purchase. You might purchase items that address a particular symptom that's bothering you, or purchase products, if different, that address the top priorities your body revealed during the testing. It's important to remember that the relationship with your practitioner is a partnership in which you receive recommendations and then decide what to do.

If your body revealed five or more reflexes in need of nutrition, however, that's far too much to correct at one time. Even if you're enthusiastic and want everything corrected right now, your practitioner will no doubt recommend that you address no more than your top three priorities. There's no point in overdoing it.

If something about your protocol feels wrong, notify your practitioner so adjustments can be made. Trust that your intuition is telling you something important, and get the help you need to find out what it is and get back on track.

Next consider how many pills you will need to take each day. This will also affect the cost. If you have a hard time taking pills, or if economic considerations are primary, you might start by addressing the top priority only. Getting that one protocol into your body will give you the nutrition that's most important now, and will also start to relieve the stress on other organs and systems that have been attempting to fill in. You will obtain the best results by taking the protocols to correct one weakness for three full months rather than by taking the protocols to correct three weaknesses for only one month.

Having selected your protocols and products, you are ready to begin the healing process.

FIFTEEN

The Process of Healing

FRESH FROM YOUR PRACTITIONER, strengthened with new information, and armed with your own personal protocol, you are ready for an important step: making a solid commitment that you will do whatever it takes to keep or regain your bone health. A strong emotional backbone in the form of personal resolve precedes a sound physical one.

Few people lose their bone health over a short period of time, and few regain it that way. Taking nutritional protocols is not like taking a pain pill or an antibiotic where you feel the difference immediately. You are undertaking the remodeling and upgrading of the basic structures that make up your bodily cells, especially those of your bones. It would be most unusual to notice major changes in a short time span. The process of regaining bone health or preventing poor bone health generally takes several visits to a health practitioner spaced three months apart.

Some people run into difficulty because they don't like to swallow pills, and the whole food concentrates and many of the herbs are in capsule or tablet form. A couple of things can help with this. Remember that you are swallowing food, not medicine. Think of your protocols as part of your meal, and include them with your breakfast, lunch, and dinner. You can also crush the tablets into a fine powder or open the capsules and sprinkle the contents into your juice or food.

Put enough pills for one meal in a small container, such as a plastic bag, so they're ready for meals away from home. In the beginning, it will take a little extra effort to get things set up, but once you get in the habit, it will be no trouble at all. Keep your long-term goal in mind. See yourself as having perfect bones and being healthy and active.

No series of protocols can promise to extend your life. But good nutrition can help prevent the foreshortening of that lifespan. Good nutrition can also support your having the best possible health while you're here. In deciding whether to follow such a program for yourself, you have to weigh the quality of your life with what you and your loved ones might stand to lose if you don't undertake this healing work. Consider the personal cost of being unable to work and requiring services to care for you; compare those costs to the cost of protocols and the quality of life they will provide you.

My bone health was so poor at one point that I had no choice but to have others take care of me. I can tell you from personal experience that even when kind, loving, and supportive people are your caregivers, it's no picnic. I'd much rather be pain free and able to function. Nobody else can take care of you the way you can.

You may feel overwhelmed at first, but it's really not that hard. You have to stick to the protocols on a daily basis, but the reward will be to find yourself growing stronger every day. This increased physical strength will in turn motivate your emotional resolve and keep you going.

Take one step at a time. When you feel like quitting, talk with supportive people—your family, practitioner, or friends. Ask them to remind you, when you feel downhearted, that healing your bones is an organic process; you didn't get this way overnight, and you won't regain perfect health overnight either.

You may wonder how long this healing process will take. The skeleton is designed to repair itself with fresh atoms every three months. The goal is to bring your body into alignment with this process. You are simply going to aid your body in doing what it already does naturally. This repair process is undertaken and completed on a three-month timetable, one layer at a time. You'll be bringing your whole body, not just your bones, closer and closer to optimum health.

How long will the entire repair process take? Bruce West, D.C., answers: "For typical sixty-five- to seventy-five-year-old women who've been osteoporotic, it's likely to be six months before strength returns and eighteen to twenty-four months before they're approaching normalcy."[1] He adds that when osteoporosis sufferers have all the factors in place—including taking the appropriate protocols, eating a proper diet with lots of raw foods, and exercising—they "can look forward to relief and feeling twenty years younger within eight to eighteen months."[2]

You will obtain the best results most quickly by working with a qualified practitioner, taking the clinical nutrition protocols that suit you, and taking them in the order that's right for you. You may not need to address all six points. Your practitioner will help you determine that.

Remember that clinical nutrition is a slow and steady process that encourages physical rebuilding, and it cannot be rushed. Nature knows how to make perfect bones; your job is to provide what is needed to support that process.

WHERE ARE THEY NOW?

This book would not be complete without returning to the people whose stories enliven its pages. For myself, since the dramatic demonstration in the airport lounge that my own bone health had come crashing down, I have taken protocols that address all points of the Six-Point Plan for Healthy Bones. This has even entailed taking some protocols more than once, as when I switched brands of vitamin C, from one that weakened my collagen fibers. Although not what I'd have chosen, this experience taught me the importance of taking whole food concentrates rather than synthetic isolates.

Before I rebuilt my body, I was exhausted and frail. Overexertion was defined by such narrow parameters as leaning over to brush my teeth in the morning, or walking to the corner and back. Now I hike and swim for hours at a time, just not too many days in a row.

I intend to continue being muscle-tested periodically and to take whatever whole food concentrates are indicated. I know from personal experience that not just my bones, but my whole body benefits. I have come to believe that this is the best health insurance there is.

We first met Carol Gieg in chapter 1, where we learned that she had suffered numerous bone fractures before the age of twenty-two. In chapter 3, she recounted her journey through the treatment options offered her by ten different physicians. Then, after meeting a muscle-testing nutritionist through her work and getting on protocols, she began by addressing weaknesses relating to Point One, connective tissue; Point Two, minerals and vitamins; and Point Three, essential fatty acids and the gallbladder support for metabolizing them. She is now working on Point Four, hormones for bones.

Carol has required longer periods on the various protocols to strengthen her systems. Some people begin to experience improvement in symptoms in three to six months, and improved bone mineral density results in one to two years. But Carol's poor bone health is one of the most long-standing kinds. Given the information available from her medical history and nutritional testing, she probably experienced follicular shutdown at an early age; follicular shutdown is a condition in which the corpus luteum of the ovum is unable to produce sufficient progesterone. It is a notoriously difficult condition to reverse.

Nonetheless, muscle testing shows considerable improvements in all her scores over the two years she has been tested. She continues a vitally active lifestyle that includes hiking, biking, and canoeing. She has suffered no additional fractures. She reports feeling that her body has some reserves now, that her hair has started growing again, and that she feels like her body could take over natural hormone production now. "Even if I don't improve from here," Carol emphasizes, "the improvement in my health is significant."

A bone mineral density (BMD) test taken soon after her improved muscle-test scores showed some improvement. However, Carol knows that BMD studies only reveal bone density, not suppleness.

We met Edith Crenshaw in chapter 3, where she was contending with the various medical options to deal with her unhealthy hip and shoulder bones. Recently Edith has been so busy taking care of her dying husband that she hasn't been able to consider the hip-replacement surgery that her doctor recommended. Her husband developed osteoporosis after being treated for prostate cancer, a treatment that involved taking a drug to lower his testosterone levels. Having seen what he has gone through with his failing bone health, it is doubtful that she will want to have the surgery. She may decide to pursue a nutritional approach instead. Her daughter is encouraging her in that direction.

Sophia Tampinelli introduced us to layers of healing in chapter 5. Not long after a practitioner tested her muscles to assess her nutritional needs, she had "a $6,000 screw" placed in her fifth metacarpal (knuckle of the hand) because she'd fractured it after falling on the street. She'd also suffered a compression fracture of T_4 (thoracic spine bone). After that, she began to realize that stress was jeopardizing her health. She has since made some major changes, including changing her employment situation. She's now had enough experience with her nutritional protocols to know what she needs to do to improve her health.

Sophia has encountered a common difficulty, however. She reports, "What I found out is that I need to be consistent about my protocol because when I start to feel better, I forget to take it, and then I slide right back. It's like antibiotics; when you feel better you don't finish the whole bottle. And when I feel bad, I feel too tired to take them. I have to will myself into taking them. At this point, I'm much more committed to doing it."

Renée Freeman, who takes care of Berle Johns, you may recall from chapter 7, told Berle that if she didn't take her nutritional protocol, she, Renée, would refuse to care for her. In 1997, Berle took the pills, which addressed Point Two, minerals and their vitamin helpers. Renée reports that following a compressed back fracture, Berle, now eighty-three, took massive doses for four months and then went on maintenance quantities. The following January, a doctor checked Berle and declared that everything was okay.

In March 1998, though, Berle fell hard, right on her hip bone. The paramedics who took her to the hospital were certain that she'd broken her hip. Since the local hospital found nothing on the X-ray, they sent her to a big-city hospital, assuming that their own equipment wasn't sophisticated enough to find the break. But there was no fracture, only bruising. Says Renée, "I just know she didn't have a fracture because of the maintenance doses she's been taking. Luckily, she's faithful about taking those pills."

From chapter 8, the miniature dachshund, Lulu, who taught me so much about the role of essential fatty acids (EFAs) in physical and emotional health, is no longer with us. After a long and active life, she finally died of old age. She remained able to take long hikes, keeping up with her brisk-walking, two-legged companions, until shortly before she died.

Once Lulu recovered from her EFA deficit, with its concomitant depression, she regained both her dynamic personality and her physical flexibility. Her recovery is an excellent example of the healing power of clinical nutrition, for she had no other agenda except to behave the way she felt. When Lulu was in pain and felt awful, she showed it directly. And when the pain was gone and she was in robust health, she demonstrated it—expressing her wants, desires, opinions, and zest for life in a variety of endearing ways.

Crystal M. shared her story about the role of gallbladder health and essential fatty acids in chapter 8. To promote her healing process, she has combined a muscle-testing approach, input from health practitioners using other approaches, products purchased over the counter, and some prescriptions recommended by physicians.

Her initial visit revealed a host of nutritional deficits affecting all six points. She's had the least health difficulty with Point One, connective tissue. For Point Two, she has taken protocols to correct mineral imbalances, especially imbalances that made her body alkaline. But the first weakness she addressed was Point Three, essential fatty acids. As you may recall, she took protocols help dissolve gallstones and to aid her bile production. Then she was able to begin metabolizing essential fatty acids, which her body desperately needed.

After raising her EFA levels, she began to address Point Four, hormone imbalances, which involved her adrenals, parathyroid, hypothalamus, thyroid gland, and sex hormone levels. As her hormonal system began to reactivate, she experienced a period of hot flashes.

Crystal's healing process has also included metabolic support for digesting proteins (Point Five), as well as addressing numerous environmental allergies, liver toxins, and parasites (Point Six).

According to bone density studies, her bone health was severely compromised before she began this healing process. Like Carol Gieg, Crystal probably experienced follicular shutdown at a young age. She was allergic to so many foods that there was very little she could eat without getting ever sicker. At one point, she weighed less than seventy pounds as a result of environmental allergies. Although she is still in the process of balancing her hormonal system, Crystal's muscle-test scores have improved significantly over a year and a half. She has continued to resist pressure by her physician to take Fosamax. As of this writing, she is about to have another bone mineral density study.

John G., you may recall from chapter 9, had low sex hormone levels as a result of surgical treatment for prostate cancer, which, his doctor said, had disappeared completely after nine weeks on nutritional protocols for yeast and virus. After this victory, John did not continue being tested, nor did he stay on any other protocols. A couple of years after his recovery from cancer, he developed Parkinson's disease; it became difficult for him to move from one room to the next, let alone get himself to an appointment in a neighboring town. Because it was so difficult for him to get to appointments and eventually even to communicate, he did not continue his sex hormone or any other protocols.

However, he was retested at age eighty-one, a few years after his surgery, and the tests revealed that he was low in essential fatty acids, his immune system was not working properly, he was very low in sex hormones, and his bone health was very poor. He did not act on these findings with any further protocols.

A few months later, John's doctor told him his cancer had recurred. A few months after that, he fell and broke his hip. During the surgery to repair his hip, John's surgeon remarked that his hip bone was like powder. His surgeon ground up the powdery bone and put it back in with wires because he thought John wouldn't survive hip replacement surgery. Afterward John fell again, which necessitated hip replacement surgery. Then he fell a third time, causing his hip joint to come out of its socket entirely and stick out under the skin. One of John's caregivers remarked that in seventeen years of taking care of people, he had never seen such unmanageable pain. John did not recover from the surgery, and died six weeks after his third fall.

John's surgeon's comment about the state of John's bone health certainly verified the muscle-test findings. John's story puts a personal face on the growing numbers of old people who fracture their hips and die. One can only wonder how the prescribed nutritional protocols might have helped his body. Would he have lived longer? Probably not. Would he have continued functioning longer and suffered less? We'll never know.

Nonetheless, his story points to the need for programs and services that would make the power of clinical nutrition easily available to the older population. If sufficient research findings were available to doctors, if insurance covered clinical nutrition, and if senior citizen care programs provided support for clinical nutritional products as well as for medications, this story may have had a different outcome. No doubt we all stand to benefit by making clinical nutrition available to our senior population, which we are all slowly joining.

Maureen Schaub is the beautician from chapters 9 and 11 whose involvement with muscle testing began when addressing the chemical poisons she is exposed to at work. The protocols, she says, put her soundly back in the game of life. The magic combination for her bones dealt with Point Six, a clean environment (toxins from work and virus); Point Four, hormones (especially thyroid, adrenals, and pituitary); and Point Three, essential fatty acids.

Checking with her a year after her first interview, she said she continues to take Parotid PMG (SP) because she continues to be exposed to chemicals at work. "I stayed with it because I kept getting headaches, and that helped keep my lungs clear of chemicals which were contributing to the headaches . . . it helps keep away the heavy feeling in my chest that I used to get."

She also continues to take Cal-Ma Plus, along with Linum B_6 to help the Cal-Ma Plus absorb into her bones. "When I stand on my feet all day at work, I don't go home at the end of the day feeling so fatigued."

Maureen says that deciding to follow through with the protocols was a learning process. "I went through a lot of difficult feelings at first, thinking it was voodoo, or a crock, because of what you're always taught. That's why my husband is skeptical. He began a protocol, started to feel better, and quit halfway through. About a year later, all his symptoms came back. Some people are skeptical and have to learn."

She explains, "I took the protocols for three months and felt a lot better, then went off them and slowly started to feel worse again. Plus, I was worried about not getting enough calcium because I can't have dairy. It is tempting to go off the protocol when you feel good; you think you don't need it, but then you start feeling bad again and realize you need to get back on it."

She adds, "I've had better success going to practitioners than doctors, so I want to stay with it. They want to work with you and get to the core of the problem, whereas with the doctor they're medicating you but not really getting to the core of it. I took my daughter [to a practitioner] before puberty when she had some illnesses, and they got to the core of it. She went through puberty with no problems, even though she'd had hives, allergic reactions to chemicals, smells, artificial colors, and preservatives. The doctors kept suppressing it with antihistamines. If she ends up getting sick now, it's something emotional. She's fifteen now, and when she gets growing pains we give her Calcium Lactate or Cal-Ma Plus and Linum B_6, whatever I have in the house, and it takes the crampiness away. Her bones test strong now, and they weren't when she was first tested. Her body was so fatigued from everything the doctors were giving her."

She adds, "My own bones are the same way, they test strong too. They were in terrible shape before, and that concerned me a lot because my grandmother had osteoporosis."

Even though she doesn't have much extra money, Maureen continues to be checked regularly for any necessary changes, and she takes her children. She says that for her, "feeling better is priceless. I would rather spend the money and know I feel good and am taking care of myself and my future. I want a healthy life in my senior years too. I don't want to go through the pain my grandmother went through."

The cost of protocols depends on how much you need to take. Whole food concentrates are usually slightly more expensive than synthetic vitamins; however, they are many times more effective and are devoid of the negative consequences of synthetics (see appendix I for details).

Maureen says she was "really sold from the time I saw my daughter getting better. When I think about how I used to feel, I don't ever want to go back. I want to move forward with my health. My health is really good now, and I want to get it even better. My goal is to get off synthetic thyroid medication entirely. My husband is still skeptical, but he's coming around I think, from seeing our experiences."

In chapter 12, Jennie deMaria wanted to be muscle-tested after reading part of the manuscript for *Perfect Bones*. Six months later, she was retested and sent this note about it: "My initial awestruck impression of muscle testing did again surface because the analysis was so immediate and exactly pertinent to my state of being. My brain was tired, my sex hormones were very low, plus I ignored my lactose intolerance at lunch, and the practitioner was able to pinpoint all of these things within five minutes even though we had not seen each other for six months."

The first testing revealed that Jennie needed to address Point Four, hormones for bones, and Point Two, minerals and their helper vitamins. After that initial test, Jennie patched together her own version of the recommended protocols from various remedies she already had at home, had heard about through friends, or could put together from dietary intake.

The second testing revealed she was still weak on adrenals and sex hormones. She remarked, "I've known my sex hormones were low, I actually have a local uncomfortableness and my sex drive is low right now, so it's not a surprise at all. I've known all along that I haven't addressed my calcium; I'm impatient with myself for ignoring it. The testing reaffirmed what I know.

"One of the many things I am thankful for in this world is second chances. Even though the analysis came through the practitioner's hands, my physical health is in my own hands. . . . I intend to share the knowledge of some of these supplements with my daughter who is nineteen and to encourage her to start using them. I may not have made deposits into a college fund for her (she is doing that herself), but I can try to make sure her calcium fund has plenty in it for her middle age. . . . I am making a concerted effort to add these supplements to my diet. . . . I hope to discern an improvement in my well-being and have another testing session to prove it in three months."

Jennie's process reminds me of what I went through initially after being tested. Like Jennie, I thought I could get some of what I needed to strengthen weak systems through diet or through synthetic products. I had to learn by trial and error, and that process taught me that whole foods are healing, but whole food concentrates are often necessary to complete the job. Jennie is doing the right thing in educating herself, making her own decisions, learning how her body responds. Luckily, she has time to do this, for she is only in middle age, and her health is fairly good.

NOW IT'S YOUR TURN

Collectively these stories demonstrate that people who continue to take their protocols, get retested, and take the next protocol for their subsequent layer of healing are constantly improving their overall health and moving further and further along in their quest for perfect bones. For Berle, the process was quick and dramatic. For Carol and Crystal, it has been slower as they deal with long-standing deficits and many layers of healing. The idea that bone health is regainable is not merely an optimistic point of view. What some have done, others can do. Their experiences also demonstrate that catching nutritional deficits early means being able to turn them around in a shorter length of time.

Once nutritional deficits are addressed, extra nutritional support may not be needed, or may be minimal. That such maintenance doses may be required has everything to do with the modern world in which we live. Our food supply is grown on leached-out, pesticide-filled soil. Then it is adulterated with fake fats, artificial sweeteners, sprays, colors, waxes, and now, genetic engineering. Governmental policies that work for the profit margins of pharmaceutical conglomerates rather than the public health can hurt us. The idea, therefore, that osteoporosis has its roots in politics is not as far-fetched as it may seem.

This modern predicament requires a modern solution. To feed yourself well, to have the vitality that should be your birthright when foods are adulterated and soils depleted, may require the addition of foods concentrated to clinical potency.

Adulterated food in combination with the modern fixation that thin is better can prove lethal for well-being, especially that of bones. A great deal of skill and know-how are required to locate, prepare, and consume foodstuffs of sufficient quality that contain real nutrients to keep one at top health. Our ancestors were able simply to reach up and pick unsullied fruits off the tree, or dig succulent tubers from a rich and fragrant earth. Their threats to survival came from tigers, bears, or warring neighbors, not from the supermarket or fast food restaurant.

Modern people have traded natural health for the relative security of homes, jobs, money, purchasing power, and the comforts provided by mass culture. Now we must learn to deal with the threats hidden within this lifestyle, particularly the bone-leaching consequences of environmental toxins and allergens, foods that are devoid of their essential nutrition, and other such stresses inherent in modern life.

A proactive stance is required. Casually consuming modern foodstuffs will not assure our health. That big, beautiful, ripe red apple looks great on the outside—but oh, what it may (or may not) contain! That local fast food restaurant may be convenient and appear inexpensive; however, making it your regular fare leads to hidden inconveniences and expenses down the line: a gradual loss of vitality, failing health, and the expenses of being unable to work.

If you feel hopeless because your mother or grandmother had osteoporosis, and you think you carry the gene, think again. Even if there were a gene for osteoporosis, the expression of all genes, including such a (theoretical) gene, is profoundly influenced by nutritional status.

And if you like some foods that are less than optimal, don't worry. Certainly the occasional consumption of fast foods can be tolerated with minimum negative effects by a healthy person. The people most likely to tolerate it are those who consistently consume a diet composed of a wide variety of fresh, whole, and generally organic foods, at least some of them raw. The key is to eat suboptimal foods rarely, and to consume little or no sugar, white flour, or refined foods. Introduction of these non-foods into the Western diet has resulted in increased dental caries, tooth sockets, bone degeneration, and skeletal deformities, a fact discovered by Westin Price, D.D.S., in his landmark study of diet and disease.[3]

For myself, I've decided to continue to be tested and to take care of weaknesses while they're still small. I want to do whatever I can to assure that I'll live until I die. I know how I feel when all my tests score a ten, and that's how I want to live if possible. If taking a few supplements a day does that for me, it's a small price to pay.

And now, what will you decide? Whatever your choice, your bones will benefit to the extent that you apply what you've learned in these pages. No doubt your healing process will be different from those stories reported here. The essential message of this book is that there *is* indeed a healing process, it is known, and there is such a process for your specific health condition.

The goal is to provide a better solution than osteoporosis to the body's need to maintain homeostatic balance. This book has covered the six essential factors that can provide that better solution. As you undergo your own bone-healing journey, you will also be making your contribution to a healthier society for us all. The information presented in this book is dedicated to that purpose.

GLOSSARY

acid: Any substance containing hydrogen that is replaceable by metals, yielding hydrogen ions as the only positively charged ions when dissolved in water.

acid-base balance: In metabolism, the balance of acid to base (alkaline ash) necessary to keep the blood neutral (slightly alkaline), between pH 7.35 and pH 7.43. Minerals found in food and stored in bone play a crucial role in keeping this balance.

acid ash diet: A diet that produces an acid ash when metabolized, often accomplished by decreasing fruits, vegetables, and milk.

alkaline: Having the reactions of a metallic hydroxide that has the property of combining with an acid to form a salt, or with an oil to form a soap.

alkaline ash diet: A diet consisting of a normal amount of protein with moderate salt restriction.

amenorrhea: The absence of menstruation.

anaphylactic shock: An acute, life-threatening form of shock resulting from an allergic reaction.

anovulatory: The cessation or suspension of ovulation.

anticholinergic: A class of drugs used to treat the side effects of several groups of prescribed drugs.

arthralgia: Joint pain.

asphyxia: A state of suspended animation due to interference with the blood's oxygen supply.

autonomic nervous system: The involuntary or self-controlling (automatic) part of the nervous system concerned with controlling involuntary functions such as glands, smooth muscle tissue, and the heart, composed of the sympathetic and parasympathetic nervous system.

calcification: Deposit in the tissues of lime salts , which are normally found in bone.

cholesterol: A crystalline substance that is soluble in fats. It is a component required to build cell membranes and sex hormones, and in certain digestive processes. It is naturally present in the brain, nervous tissue, blood, liver (where about four-fifths of it is manufactured), and bile. It is the largest component of gallstones.

collagen: A substance existing in various tissues of the body, as in the white fibers of connective tissue. It is the protein prepared from connective tissue (such as tendons) from which gelatin is made.

connective tissue: That which connects or binds together; one of the four main tissues of the body. After embryonic connective tissue becomes adult, it is found in vascular tissues such as blood and lymph, fibrous tissues, cartilage, and bone. These tissues support bodily structures, bind parts together, store food, and play a role in blood formation and some defensive mechanisms.

C-section (cesarean section): The surgical removal of the fetus from the womb.

co-factors: Additional nutrients and enzymes needed to completely metabolize and use a given nutrient.

collagen: An elastic living matrix made up of protein.

corticosteroids: Hormones produced by the adrenal glands.

desiccated: Designating products made from a concentrate of the whole gland, as in desiccated adrenal or desiccated parathyroid.

ecosanoid: Pertaining to essential fatty acids.

ectoderm: The outer layer of cells in a developing embryo, from which develop skin structures (including the gut), the nervous system, organs of special sense (nose, eye, and ear), the pineal gland, and part of the pituitary and suprarenal glands.

electrical charge: The quantity of positive, negative, or neutral energy present in a tissue, expressed chemically as valence. It is caused by the motion of protons, neutrons, and electrons, and it manifests as attraction, repulsion, or magnetic forces.

endocrine: Organs or glands that secrete substances such as hormones.

endoderm: The innermost layer of cells in a developing embryo from which arise the epithelium of the digestive tract and its associated glands and the respiratory organs, bladder, vagina, and urethra.

enzyme: An organic compound capable of breaking down a substance into its component parts.

ester: A compound formed by combining an organic acid with alcohol. It often has a fruity or flowery smell.

fatty acids: A variety of organic acids from which fats or oils are made. Essential ones are those whose absence in the diet leads to loss of weight, eczematous skin conditions, and kidney disorders.

follicle: A small secretory sac or cavity such as those found in the ovary or thyroid, or oil-producing ones in the skin.

free radical: An electrically charged atom that attacks body cells. It creates oxidative stress and can cause cells to lose function and structure, and can eventually destroy the cell.

hormone: A chemical substance originating in an organ or gland, which is conveyed through the blood to another part of the body, stimulating it to increased functional activity and increased secretion.

hydroxyapatite: The crystals in bone made of collagen and mineral deposits in combination.

hypogonadal: Low sex-hormone producing (referring to gonads).

hypertension: High blood pressure, often the result of narrowing of the blood vessels, due in part to calcium formation on the vessel walls and sometimes related to magnesium deficiency.

hysterectomy: The surgical removal of the uterus, sometimes includes oophorectomy also, which is removal of the ovaries.

keratin: A protein found in hair and nails.

ketogenic: Promoting the production of ketones, which are breakdown products of the fat-burning process.

ligament: A band or sheet of strong, fibrous connective tissue connecting the ends of bones, serving to bind them together and to facilitate or limit motion, to support visceral organs, or to connect cartilage, muscles, and other structures.

mesoderm: The middle primary germ layer of the developing embryo from which arise all connective tissues: muscular, skeletal, circulatory, lymphatic, and urogenital systems and the linings of the body cavities.

micronized progesterone: An exact chemical duplicate of the progesterone that the human body produces. Derived from extracts of yams and soybeans.

mineral: "Any class of substances occurring in nature, usually comprising inorganic substances, as quartz, feldspar, etc., of definite chemical composition and usually of definite crystal structure, but sometimes also including rocks formed by these substances as well as certain natural products of organic origin, as asphalt, coal, etc. Any substance that is neither animal nor vegetable." *(Random House Dictionary of the English Language).*

nutraceutical: A food product or herb that has been changed slightly in its molecular structure, making it possible to patent the product.

oophorectomy: The surgical removal of the ovaries.

osmosis: A process that allows for elements contained in solution to pass through cell membranes so they can be used for cell metabolism or to carry out products of elimination.

osteitis deformans: A chronic, slowly progressive bone disorder, in which an initial phase of decalcification and softening is followed by calcium deposition with thickening, abnormal architecture, and deformity. Also called Paget's disease.

osteoblast: Bone cell that forms new bone.

osteoclast: Bone cell that resorbs old bone.

osteocyte: A living bone cell that can become an osteoclast or an osteoblast.

osteogenesis: The formation and development of bone that takes place in connective tissue or cartilage.

osteogenesis imperfecta: A Latin term referring to the imperfect formation and development of bone due to defective collagen, causing bones to fracture easily. Some experts consider it a genetic disorder, others a nutritional one relating to protein in connective tissue.

osteoid: The noncellular collagenous matrix of bone.

osteopenia: A value for bone mineral density (BMD) that lies between –1 and –2.5 standard deviations below the young adult mean value. This finding is interpreted as early-stage bone loss.

osteoporosis: The diminished structural integrity of the skeleton, including decreased bone mass, involving loss of both mineral and protein matrix components of bone. Also, a value for bone mineral density (BMD) that lies more than –2.5 standard deviations below the young adult mean value.

osteomyelitis: A bone infection resulting from pyogenic (pus-producing) microorganisms.

otosclerosis: Progressive deafness due to the formation of spongy bone around the stapes bone in the ear.

perimenopausal: The time surrounding menopause when many hormone changes occur.

pH: A symbol used to express the degree of acidity or alkalinity of a solution. Neutral pH is 7; stomach juices are often 1.0 to 1.3; blood plasma is 7.3 to 7.5.

phagocytosis: Ingestion and digestion of bacteria and particles by phagocytes, a type of cell that keeps the body free of invaders and debris.

prodromal: The initial phase of getting sick, especially with an infection.

prostaglandin: A substance resembling a hormone that regulates various body processes, especially those related to inflammation.

prothrombin: A chemical substance in circulating blood that interacts with calcium salts to produce thrombin, which helps to clot blood once it is shed.

phylogenetic: Concerning the development of a race or group.

phytochemicals: Whole nutrients contained in plants.

phytoestrogen: Plant sources of estrogen or plant substances from which estrogen is made.

precursor: A nutrient in a form that precedes another form.

preeclampsia: A toxic condition of pregnancy with high blood pressure that increases headaches, albuminuria, and swelling of the lower extremities.

premenopausal: Before the cessation of menses.

progestational agent: Any one of several chemical substances that have the effect of progesterone. They are usually synthetic and are used in birth control pills.

progesterone: A natural steroid hormone found in the corpus luteum (the part of the ovarian follicle that makes progesterone) and the placenta. It is responsible for changes in uterine lining (endometrium) in the second half of the menstrual cycle preparatory for implantation of the newly fertilized egg (blastocyst), development of maternal placenta after implantation, and development of mammary glands.

Progestins: A term used to cover a large group of synthetic drugs that have a progesterone-like effect on the uterus. They are used in medications like oral contraceptives. Some are synthetically derived from the male hormone, testosterone, or chemically modified from natural progesterone. Synthetic Progestins can inhibit ovulation, thus suppressing the body's output of its own hormone, progesterone.

progestogens: Any natural or synthetic hormonal substance that produces effects similar to those due to progesterone.

protocol: A plan to follow consisting of a series of steps, a regimen. A clinical nutrition protocol includes a list of products along with instructions for taking them over a length of time, usually three months.

protomorphogen (PMG): The biological template for organs, made of complexes of nucleoprotein molecules, a phosphorus backbone, and a mineral substrate with as many as ninety trace minerals.

resorption: The process by which a substance is dissolved or eliminated.

subluxation: A partial or incomplete dislocation of a bone.

tetany: Muscle spasms often related to parathyroid deficiency, emotional excitement, or infectious fevers.

tocopherols: One of several alcohols that comprise the dietary factor known as vitamin E. They are found in wheat germ oil, lettuce, spinach leaves, egg yolk, and other sources.

transdermal: Through the skin, as in transdermal creams that deliver medications or herbs through the skin.

transfatty acid: A fatty acid chain having a pair of identical atoms or groups on the opposite sides of two atoms linked by a double bond. They are known to raise levels of "bad" cholesterol and decrease "good" cholesterol. They are found in many baked and fried foods. Studies suggest that the more transfatty acids consumed, the greater the risk of developing heart disease and premature death.

triglyceride: The form in which fat is stored in the body when excess calories are consumed. It consists of three fatty acids attached to a glycerol molecule.

valence: A measure of the combining power or relative capacity of an atom to interact with a biological building block (substrate).

Why Use Whole Food Concentrates?

WHOLE FOOD CONCENTRATES contain essential food factors known by science (and some factors science has yet to discover) that nature has always provided, including trace minerals, enzymes, and other factors such as coenzymes and antioxidants. For example, one B vitamin (B_4) is officially recognized in Great Britain but not in the United States. Synthetic vitamin C (ascorbic acid), which is made by boiling corn syrup and sulfuric acid together, is known to cause genetic damage at a dosage of 500 milligrams a day for six weeks. Natural vitamin E is a complex with eight parts; synthetic vitamin E sold over the counter contains one to four chemical imitations of the eight natural parts.

- Ingesting one isolated part of a vitamin complex requires the body to borrow the other, missing factors from its own stores, thus creating a physical deficiency of the other factors over time.
- Without the trace mineral activators found in whole food vitamins, the vitamin fails in its metabolic function.
- Synthetics are extracted and fractionated. They contain isolated chemical fragments that are dead chemical models of living foods.

- Synthetics can fool the body into thinking they're the real things, thus occupying the sites where the real thing would be taken up and utilized, thereby blocking the action of the real food.
- Synthetic vitamins can prevent death on a short-term basis, but not promote life. Whole food concentrates promote life.
- Natural vitamin complexes are functional mechanisms that work together synergistically to produce a result that is not revealed by chemical analysis of its components.
- The "aliveness" of whole food concentrates and the relative "deadness" of synthetic vitamins cannot by seen by chemical analysis, but can be seen by the process of chromatography, which is not currently used by manufacturers or the government to assess the merits of a product.
- With whole foods and whole food concentrates, the body can selectively absorb what it needs and choose to excrete what it doesn't need. With synthetic vitamins, the body loses this choice; it is required to process this chemical somehow, which can lead to chemical imbalances or toxic overdoses.
- The body treats all synthetic vitamins as toxic, and its attempt to process them can result in imbalances that are worse than the deficiency they were supposed to correct.
- The body requires vitamins in two forms (called dextro-rotatory and levo-rotatory, or right-handed and left-handed). Synthetics provide only one form, but occupy both sites producing chemical "mistakes" in the cells in which they are used.

Why Use Whole Plant Extracts of Whole Herbs?

THE MOST EFFECTIVE HERBAL PRODUCTS begin with evaluation of a sample from the field. Starting with herbs of known good quality, as determined by chemical assay, this ensures that:

- The right species of herb is used. Many herbal products use the wrong species of herb for its intended benefit.
- Each batch of herbs is unadulterated. Some herbs have been fluffed or blended with other herbs, a fact that often remains unknown even to herb vendors because they did not evaluate the herbs.
- The herbs used in the product are demonstrated to be full spectrum, containing the full range of active ingredients. Many herbal products sold on the market are not.
- The product will contain the full spectrum, not only of constituents, but also of activity. Single-constituent extract products demonstrate a limited-spectrum activity.
- The herbs used to make the product are free of contaminants, such as pesticides, herbicides, extraneous matter, heavy metals, aflatoxins, microbes, or radiation. Many herbal products carry one or more of these contaminants.
- The right part of the plant will be employed—the one that contains the active principles; for example, the root and not the leaves. Many products use the wrong plant part.

- The batch of product contains *complexes* of herbs; in other words, it contains all the ingredients that make the plant effective (active principles) in the whole plant matrix, as nature made the plant, not altered chemically or biologically.

The ideal manufacturing process:

- begins with a quality-assurance process (including tests for color, aroma, texture, content of specified actives, Thin Layer Chromatography fingerprinting, gas chromatography, microbiological levels, the amount of extraneous matter, pesticides and herbicides, heavy metals, aflatoxins, and radiation levels).
- mills at low temperature to protect active components.
- follows detailed procedures describing when to add each component, to guarantee a highly potent product.
- uses cold processing because thermal energy in the processing breaks chemical bonds; although some bonds will reattach, the herb would be rendered less effective.
- uses water purified by reverse osmosis.
- is carried out in a manufacturing complex using pharmaceutical-standard air filtration, which has a higher standard than other methods.
- requires the product to pass stringent testing and meet standardized criteria at every phase.
- requires the product to meet British pharmacopoeia standards (most are food grade only).
- produces tablets tested for disintegration, friability, weight uniformity, and active constituents.

Only MediHerb of Australia meets all these criteria, which is why health professionals use these powerful products.

Common Symptoms of Estrogen Dominance

"OVER 80 PERCENT OF BREAST CANCERS are caused by estrogen dominance," said John Lee, M.D., in a telephone interview in May 2002. Estrogen dominance has many causes, including the changes of perimenopause and menopause, contraceptive use, hormone replacement therapy, and poor nutrition. The following are common symptoms of estrogen dominance, according to Robert Gottesman, M.D., and John Lee, M.D.

- Acceleration of the aging process
- Allergies, including asthma, hives, rashes, sinus congestion
- Autoimmune disorders such as lupus erythematosis and thyroiditis and possibly Sjoegren's disease
- Bloating
- Breast cancer
- Breast tenderness
- Cervical dysplasia
- Cold hands and feet as a symptom of thyroid dysfunction
- Decreased sex drive
- Depression with anxiety or agitation
- Dry eyes
- Early onset of menstruation

- Endometriosis
- Fat gain, especially around the abdomen, hips, and thighs
- Fatigue
- Fibrocystic breasts
- Gallbladder disease
- Hair loss
- Headaches
- Hypoglycemia
- Inability to focus
- Increased blood clotting (increasing risk of strokes)
- Infertility
- Insomnia
- Irregular menstrual periods
- Irritability
- Memory loss
- Miscarriage
- Mood swings
- Osteoporosis
- Ovarian cancer
- PMS
- Poor sleep or disturbed sleep
- Premenopausal bone loss
- Prostate cancer
- Sluggish metabolism
- Uterine cancer
- Uterine fibroids
- Water retention or bloating

Sources

Standard Process and MediHerb
For referral to a practitioner:
800-558-8740
email: info@standardprocess.com

For Standard Process and Mediherb
  products in the United States:
1200 West Royal Lee Drive
Palmyra, WI 53156
800-848-5061
fax: 414-495-2512

For Standard Process products from
  non–U.S. locations:
Standard Process of Northern
  California
6201 Doyle Street, #A
Emeryville, CA 94608
510-597-9100
contact: Justin Toal

For MediHerb in Australia:
P.O. Box 713
Warwick, Qld. 4370
Australia
+61 7 4661 0700
fax: +61 7 4661 0788

For MediHerb in Denmark:
Danske Urte-Central
Dronningensgade 60
7000 Fredericia
Denmark
+ 45 7591 1811
fax: +45 7591 3636
contact: Karenmai Pedersen

For MediHerb in New Zealand:
Professional Herb Services Ltd.
P.O. Box 9344
Addington, Christchurch
New Zealand
+64 3 338 8166
fax: +64 3 338 8146
contact: Paul Mitchell

**Specific Sources Mentioned in the
  Book**
For Dr. Michael Dobbins' videotape
  library:
DPG Video
5960 S. Land Park Drive, #143
Sacramento, CA 95822

For Bernard Jensen and Mark
Anderson's *Empty Harvest:*
Standard Process West
P.O. Box 270547
Fort Collins, CO 80527-0547
800-321-9807
Contact for a signed copy.

For Dr. Royal Lee's lectures:
Selene River Press
800-321-9807

For information on hormone
disruptors, search:
Environmental Protection Agency
www.epa.gov
World Wildlife Fund Canada
www.wwfcanada.org

For natural progesterone supplements:
The Women's International Pharmacy
2 Marsh Court
Madison, WI 53718
800-279-5708
www.womensinternational.com

For salivary hormone testing for
health professionals only:
Great Smokies Diagnostic Laboratory
63 Zillicoa Street
Asheville, NC 28801
800-522-4762
fax: 828-252-9303
email: cs@gsdl.com
www.gsdl.com

For salivary hormone testing for all
consumers:
ZRT Laboratory
1815 NW 169th Place, Suite 5050
Beaverton, OR 97006
503-466-2445
Hormone hotline: 503-466-9166
fax: 503-466-1636
email: info@salivatest.com
www.salivatest.com
Six hormone tests are available; they
are $30 each as of this writing.

For information on pollution in your
area, enter your zip code at:
www.scorecard.org
Service provided by the
Environmental Defense Fund.

**General Health and Nutrition
Sources**
The American Association of
Naturopathic Physicians
3201 New Mexico Avenue NW
Suite 350
Washington, DC 20016
866-538-2267
www.naturopathic.org

*The American Journal of Clinical
Nutrition*
www.faseb.org/ajcn

The American Society for Clinical
Nutrition
www.faseb.org/ascn

Citizens for Health, Defending Your
  Right to Choose
P. O. Box 2260
Boulder, CO 80306
800-357-2211
www.citizens.org
For more about your right to know
  personal health care information.

Health Alert Newsletter
5 Harris Court, N6
Monterey, CA 93940
408-372-2103
www.healthalert.com

International Foundation for Nutrition
  and Health
3963 Mission Boulevard
San Diego, CA 92109
858-488-8932
fax: 858-488-2566
www.ifnh.org
Contact for a catalog of books and
  materials on nutrition.

Men's Health Consulting
Will Courtnay, Ph.D., L.C.S.W.
2811 College Avenue, Suite 1
Berkeley, CA 94705-2167
800-WELL-MEN
www.menshealth.org
Provides education to health
  professionals, work sites, and
  colleges addressing behaviors and
  beliefs that damage men's health,
  including beliefs about manhood.

National Women's Health Network
514 10th Street NW, #400
Washington, DC 20004
202-628-7814
www.womenshealthnetwork.org

Price-Pottenger Nutrition Foundation
P.O. Box 2614
La Mesa, CA 91943-2614
800-FOODS4U
www.price-pottenger.org
Professional and lay memberships.
  Physician referral lists for three
  states of your choice for $6.

ENDNOTES

Every effort has been made to ensure the accuracy of the following sources, but some websites may no longer be current due to the constantly changing nature of the World Wide Web. If you spot any error, please feel free to contact the publisher with the correct information.

PART ONE

Chapter 1

1. National Institutes of Health Osteoporosis and Related Bone Diseases National Resource Center, "Bone Basics for Men of All Ages" (Washington, DC: National Institutes of Health, June 1996 and July 1997): 1.

2. James Balch, M.D., and Phyllis A. Balch, C.N.C., *Prescription for Nutritional Healing,* 2nd edition (Garden City Park, NY: Avery, 1997), 413.

3. "Science Matters," *Ukiah Daily Journal* (March 30, 1997): A-11.

4. Wyeth-Ayerst Laboratories advertisement, *USA Weekend* (September 26–28, 1997): 11.

5. Wyeth-Ayerst Laboratories Prempro advertisement, *USA Weekend* (September 19–21, 1997): 24–25.

6. Gail Sheehy, *New Passages: Mapping Your Life across Time* (New York: Random House, 1995), 200.

7. Clare Dover, *Osteoporosis* (London, England: Ward Lock in conjunction with the National Osteoporosis Society, 1994), 11.

8. Osteoporosis Australia, "About Osteoporosis," available at www.osteoporosis.org.au/html/aboutosteomain.php.

9. Osteoporosis in Men, "In-Depth Report on the State of Osteoporosis in

Men," available at www.geocities.com/HotSprings/8741/
osteoporosis_in_men.html.

10. Royal Lee, D.D.S., *Therapeutic Food Manual* (no publication date), 70.

11. Ibid.

12. Bernard Jensen and Mark Anderson, *Empty Harvest: Understanding the Link between Our Food, Our Immunity, and Our Planet* (Garden City Park, NY: Avery, 1990), 10, 24, 47.

13. John Lee, M.D., *Natural Progesterone: The Multiple Roles of a Remarkable Hormone* (Sebastopol, CA: BLL Publishing, 1993), 37.

14. Sources include the National Osteoporosis Foundation; *The Journal of the American Dietetic Association; The Johns Hopkins Medical Newsletter; The Mount Sinai Journal of Medicine; The Medical Data Exchange (MDX);* Mae Tinklenberg, M.S., R.N., "Healthwatch," *NurseWeek* (June 24, 1996): 21; "Bone Up to Prevent Osteoporosis," *Energy Times* (January 1997): Women's Health, 18; and John Lee, M.D., *Natural Progesterone.*

15. Valerie Peck, M.D., "Depression-Osteoporosis Link Found," *Ukiah Daily Journal* (March 30, 1997): A-11.

Chapter 2

1. Dover, *Osteoporosis,* 13.

2. Health Information for African American Women, "African American Women," available at www.4woman.gov/minority/index.cfm?page=172.

3. Peter D'Adamo, N.D., *Eat Right for Your Type* (New York: Riverhead/ Putnam, 1996), 8.

4. "Calcium: Beneficial to Bones and More," *Healthy Cell News* (spring/ summer 1996): 17.

5. B. L. Riggs and L. J. Melton, "The Prevention and Treatment of Osteoporosis," *New England Journal of Medicine,* vol. 327, no. 9 (August 27, 1992): 620–27.

6. "Calcium: Beneficial to Bones and More," 17.

7. Dover, *Osteoporosis,* 8, 10.

8. D. A. Versendaal, D.C., Ph.D., author's interview, January 24, 1998.

9. National Institutes of Health Osteoporosis and Related Bone Diseases National Resource Center, "Fast Facts on Osteoporosis," available at www.osteo.org/osteolinks.asp.

10. Lisa Lanucci, "Bone Power," *Energy Times* (May 1997): 59.

11. Jean Carper, "Calcium: Not for Women Only," *USA Weekend* (March 27–29, 1998): 15.

12. National Osteoporosis Foundation, "Men with Osteoporosis, in Their Own Words" (Washington, DC: National Osteoporosis Foundation, 1997).

13. National Institutes of Health Osteoporosis and Related Bone Diseases

National Resource Center, "Fast Facts on Osteoporosis," available at www.osteo.org/osteolinks.asp.

14. Ibid.

15. Dover, *Osteoporosis*, 8.

16. Ibid., 36.

17. Ibid., 33.

18. Balch and Balch, *Prescription for Nutritional Healing*, 413.

19. Horace B. Deets, "AARP's Realignment," AARP Perspectives, *Modern Maturity* (November/December 1997): 1.

20. PR Newswire, "Journal of the American Medical Association Reports: Calcium during Pregnancy Could Save Lives," available at www.kidsource.com/kidsource/content/news/calcium.4.9.html.

21. Eric Barefield, "Osteoporosis-Related Hip Fractures Cost $13 Billion to $18 Billion Yearly: Moving toward Healthier Diets," *Food Review* (January 13, 1996).

Chapter 3

1. Jerry Green, J.D., "The Health Care Contract: A Model for Sharing Responsibility," *Somatics*, vol. 3, no. 4 (1982).

2. Alan Gaby, M.D., *Preventing and Reversing Osteoporosis: Every Woman's Essential Guide* (Rocklin, CA: Prima Publishing, 1994), ix.

3. John Lee, M.D., "Osteoporosis Reversal: The Role of Progesterone," *The International Clinical Nutrition Review*, vol. 10, no. 3 (July 1990): 384.

4. Arturo Corces, M.D., summarized remarks at conferences of the National Institutes of Health Osteoporosis and Related Bone Diseases National Resource Center, June 1996 and July 1997.

5. Menopause and Beyond, "Aspects of Osteoporosis," available at www.oxford.net/~tishy/osteo.html.

6. John Lee, *Natural Progesterone*, 84.

7. J. C. Prior, "Progesterone As a Bone-Trophic Hormone," *Endocrine Reviews*, vol. 11, no. 2 (May 1990): 386–400.

8. Kerri Bodmer, "Editronate and Osteoporosis," *Women's Health Letter*, vol. 7, no. 5 (May 1998): 6.

9. Kerri Bodmer, "Healthy Body, Healthy Bones," *Women's Health Letter*, vol. 6, no. 7 (July 1998): 1.

10. Reuters, "Self-Administered U.S. Test Aims to Measure Bone Loss," *The Industry Standard* (August 16, 2001), available at www.thestandard.com/wire/0%2C2231%2C26065%2C00.html.

11. Available at www.osteometer.com/aboutosteometer.htm.

12. "High Bone Density Doesn't Always Protect Women from Fractures," *Great Smokies Connection*, vol. 13, no. 11.

13. Kerri Bodmer, "Women's Health News: The Latest Healing Breakthroughs for Women," *Women's Health Letter* (summer 1999): 8.

14. John Lee, *Natural Progesterone*, 42.

15. Kerri Bodmer with Nan Kathryn Fuchs, *Stop Breast Cancer before It Happens* (Atlanta, GA: Soundview Publications, Inc., 1997), 16.

16. William Campbell Douglass, M.D., "Say Goodbye to Illness," *Health Breakthroughs* (fall 1997): 12.

17. American Pharmaceutical Association, via a grant from Sandoz Pharmaceuticals Corporation and the National Osteoporosis Foundation, advertisement, January 1998.

18. John Robbins, *Reclaiming Our Health: Exploding the Medical Myth and Embracing the Source of True Healing* (Tiburon, CA: H. J. Kramer, 1996), 151.

19. Eric Fidler, "Study: Osteoporosis Drug Lowers Risk of Breast Cancer," *Ukiah Daily Journal* (September 5, 1999): B-3.

20. John Lee, M.D., author's interview, May 2002.

21. Merck Pharmaceuticals advertisement for Fosamax; and Tinklenberg, "Healthwatch," 24.

22. John Lee, *Natural Progesterone*, 49.

23. John Lee, M.D., "Osteoporosis Reversal: The Role of Progesterone," *The International Clinical Nutrition Review* (July 1990): 389.

24. John Lee, author's interview, May 2002

25. Wyeth-Ayerst Laboratories advertisement, *USA Weekend* (September 26–28, 1997): 11.

26. Michelle Paslucci. "Researchers Cancel Study After Proving Prempro's Risks," *NurseWeek* (August 12, 2002): 8.

27. Gaby, *Preventing and Reversing Osteoporosis*, 139.

28. "ERT/HRT Market Continues to Grow," *Drug Store News* (May 17, 1999).

29. Gaby, *Preventing and Reversing Osteoporosis*, 234.

30. Mary Ann Hellinghausen, Leigh Morgan, and Valeria J. Nelson, *NurseWeek* (June 23, 1997).

31. G. E. Abraham and H. Grewal, "A Total Dietary Program Emphasizing Magnesium Instead of Calcium: Effect on the Mineral Density of Cacaneous Bone in Postmenopausal Women on Hormonal Therapy," *Journal of Reproductive Medicine*, vol. 35, no. 5 (May 1990): 503–7. Available at www.mdschoice.com/text/abstracts/Magnesium/magosteo.htm.

32. Kerri Bodmer, "Don't Let New Fosamax Study Fool You," *Women's Health Letter*, vol. 7, no. 4 (April 1998): 6.

33. Bodmer, "Editronate and Osteoporosis," 6.

34. *Taber's Cyclopedic Medical Dictionary*, 8th edition (Philadelphia: F. A. David Company, 1960), 1–23.

35. Bodmer, "Healthy Body, Healthy Bones," 1.

36. John Lee, M.D., author's interview, March 7, 2002.

37. John Lee, M.D., lecture presented at the Graton Women's Club, Graton, CA, 2000.

38. Gaby, *Preventing and Reversing Osteoporosis,* 233.

39. John Lee, M.D., with Virginia Hopkins, *What Your Doctor May Not Tell You about Menopause: The Breakthrough Book on Natural Progesterone* (New York: Warner, 1996), 169.

40. Tinklenberg, "Healthwatch," 21.

41. Gaby, *Preventing and Reversing Osteoporosis,* 234.

42. Tinklenberg, "Healthwatch," 21.

43. John Lee, *Natural Progesterone,* 68.

44. Gaby, *Preventing and Reversing Osteoporosis,* 235.

45. Michael Dobbins, D.C., "Effective Nutrition Therapy," a professional seminar, Berkeley, CA, February 28, 1998.

46. Adam Marcus, "A New Strategy for Fighting Osteoporosis," *Johns Hopkins Magazine Online* (June 1997), available at www.jhu.edu/~jhumag/ 0697web/health.html.

47. Depression Info Center, "Bone Mineral Density Decreased in Patients with Major Depression," available at www.mhsource.com/depression/ bone.html.

48. Alan S. Levin, M.D., J.D., author's interview, May 1998.

49. "Human Bone Grown outside the Body," *BBC News Online* (October 18, 2000), available at http://news.bbc.co.uk/low/english/health/ newsid_976000/976711.stm.

50. IMS Health (a research firm that tracks prescription drug data).

51. Deborah Baurac, "Joint Exchange," *Modern Maturity* (September/October 1997): 68.

52. Jason Theodosakis, M.D., M.S., M.P.H., Brenda Adderly, M.H.A., and Barry Fox, Ph.D., *The Arthritis Cure* (New York: St. Martin's Press, 1997), 3.

53. Gaby, *Preventing and Reversing Osteoporosis,* 40.

54. Balch and Balch, *Prescription for Nutritional Healing,* 416.

55. Gaby, *Preventing and Reversing Osteoporosis,* 40.

56. Balch and Balch, *Prescription for Nutritional Healing,* 416.

57. Gaby, *Preventing and Reversing Osteoporosis,* v (Jonathan Wright's introduction).

58. Jean Barilla, M.S., "Rx for Health Care," *The Physicians Newsletter: Health through Nutrition,* vol. 2, no. 1 (April 1997): 1.

59. Eric Rose, M.D., "Pharmaceutical Marketing in the United States: A Critical Analysis" (1997), available at http://faculty.washington.edu/momus/ pharm.htm.

60. Kerri Bodmer, "Update on Calcium Channel Blockers," *Women's Health Letter,* vol. 7, no. 5 (May 1998): 5.

61. Douglass, "Say Goodbye to Illness," 12.

62. Dean Black, "Artful Science: Documenting the Chiropractic Experience," Parker College (unpublished article), 1996), 1. Quoted in Peter Clecak, Ph.D., "Giving Patients 'Reasonable Counsel': The Case of Contact Reflex Analysis" (unpublished article): 1.

63. Barbara Griggs, *Green Pharmacy* (Rochester, VT: Healing Arts Press, 1997), 243.

64. Ibid., 238.

65. Gaby, *Preventing and Reversing Osteoporosis,* xiv.

Chapter 4

1. Green, "The Health Care Contract."

2. Dobbins, "Effective Nutrition Therapy."

3. Royal Lee, "The Systemic Causes of Dental Caries," paper presented at Marquette University, December 1923.

4. Westin Price, D.D.S., *Nutrition and Physical Degeneration* (La Mesa, CA: Price-Pottenger Nutritional Foundation, 1939), 34.

5. Dobbins, "Effective Nutrition Therapy."

6. Mary Jane Mack, R.N., author's interview, April 28, 1998.

7. Judith DeCava, M.S., C.C.N., *The Real Truth about Vitamins and Antioxidants,* Health Science Series #5 (Columbus, GA: Brentwood Academic Press, 1996), 209, 216–221.

8. Fred Ulan, D.C., C.C.N., and Lester Bryman, D.C., "CRA New Client Orientation," *CRA Collector's Edition* (1996), 2–3.

9. MPI NuPro, "Natural vs. Synthetic (Is Natural Better?)," *The NuPro Therapist,* vol. 2, no. 2.

10. Dobbins, "Effective Nutrition Therapy."

11. Ibid.

12. Ibid.

13. Bruce West, D.C., "Am I Biased?" *Health Alert,* vol. 14, no. 9 (September 1997): 1.

14. Ibid.

15. *The Training Session: Introduction to Standard Process.*

16. Dobbins, "Effective Nutrition Therapy."

17. Peter D'Adamo, N.D., *4 Your Type: Custom Supplements Made Right 4 Your Type by Dr. Peter D'Adamo,* product catalog, 2002: 5.

18. Simon Mills and Kerry Bone, *Principles and Practice of Phytotherapy: Modern Herbal Medicine* (Edinburgh, Scotland: Churchill Livingstone, 2000).

19. Bruce West, D.C., "Allergic to Everything," *Health Alert,* vol. 14, no. 5 (May 1997): 3–4.

20. Bruce West, D.C., author's interview, January 1999.

21. Ibid.

22. Mack, author's intereview.

Chapter 5

1. Gaby, *Preventing and Reversing Osteoporosis,* vi (Jonathan Wright's introduction).

2. Dobbins, "Effective Nutrition Therapy."

PART TWO

Chapter 6

1. John Lee, *Natural Progesterone,* 55.

2. Dobbins, "Effective Nutrition Therapy."

3. *The Training Session: Introduction to Standard Process,* 16.

4. Royal Lee, *Therapeutic Food Manual.*

5. Lee Vagt, D.C., author's interview, June 1996.

6. Gaby, *Preventing and Reversing Osteoporosis,* 95.

7. Susan E. Brown, Ph.D., *Better Bones, Better Body* (New Canaan, CT: Keats Publishing Company, 1996), 89.

8. Gaby, *Preventing and Reversing Osteoporosis,* 31.

9. Ibid., 96.

10. Bruce West, D.C., "High Dose Vitamin C Causes Problems," *Health Alert,* vol. 15, no. 9 (July 1998), 8.

11. Lisa Lanucci, "Bone Power," *Energy Times* (January 1997): 18.

12. Balch and Balch, *Prescription for Nutritional Healing,* 21.

13. Ibid., 20.

14. *The Training Session: Introduction to Standard Process,* 13.

15. Ibid.

16. Dobbins, "Effective Nutrition Therapy."

17. Michael Murray, N.D. "The *True* Arthritis Cure," in *Arthritis Counselor,* special edition (1997): 11.

18. "Sulfur: An Ancient Nutrient Needed Now, More Than Ever Before," *American Council on Collaborative Medicine,* vol. 4, no. 3 (March 1998): 1.

19. Michael Colgan, Ph.D., *Hormonal Health: Nutritional and Hormonal Strategies for Emotional Well-Being and Intellectual Longevity* (Vancouver, Canada: Apple Publishing, 1996), 117.

20. *Standard Process Clinical Reference Guide,* 25.

21. Dan Newell, C.N., author's interview, July 1999.

22. Dobbins, "Effective Nutrition Therapy."

23. Newell, author's interview.

24. Vagt, author's interview.

25. J. Masquelier, et al., "Stabilization of Collagen by Procanidolic Oligomers," *Acta Therapeutica*, 7 (1981): 101–105.

26. *The Training Session: Introduction to Standard Process*, 17.

27. Raymond D. Schmidt. "A Treatment for Leprosy," *Health Journal*, vol. 21, no. 3: 1.

28. Vagt, Ibid.

29. Vagt, author's interview.

30. *MediHerb Professional Review*, no. 59 (August 1997).

31. B. Brinkhaus, et al., "*Centella Asiatica* in Traditional and Modern Phytomedicine: A Pharmacological and Clinical Profile," *Perfusion*, vol. 11 (1998): 508–20.

32. F. Bonte, et al., "Influence of Asiatic Acid, Madecassic Acid, and Asiaticoside on Human Collagen I Synthesis," *Planta Medica*, vol. 60, no. 2 (1994): 133–35.

33. N. Blumenkrantz, et al., "Effect of (+)-Catechin on Connective Tissue," *Scandinavian Journal of Rheumatology*, 7 (1978): 55–60.

34. *MediHerb Professional Review*, no. 59 (August 1997).

Chapter 7

1. Dover, *Osteoporosis*, 48.

2. Dobbins, "Effective Nutrition Therapy."

3. "Calcium: Beneficial to Bones and More," 17.

4. *Standard Process Clinical Reference Guide*, 15.

5. Dobbins, "Effective Nutrition Therapy."

6. Bruce West, D.C., "Diseases of Calcium Metabolism," *Health Alert*, vol. 15, no. 5: 5.

7. Sharon Bortz, M.S., R.D., "Boning Up on Calcium," *Redwood Health Club Newsletter* (September 1997): 1.

8. Mildred Jackson, N.D., and Terri Teague, *The Handbook of Alternatives to Chemical Medicine* (Oakland, CA: Lawton-Teague, 1975), 144.

9. Bob LeRoy, R.D., "Major Study Results Challenge Claims for Dairy," *Vegetarian Voice* (fall 1997): 19.

10. Royal Lee, D.D.S., talk for the American Academy of Nutrition Society, Long Beach, CA, April 1955.

11. Balch and Balch, *Prescription for Nutritional Healing*, 414.

12. Ibid., 415.

13. Gaby, *Preventing and Reversing Osteoporosis,* 101.

14. Elizabeth Sutherland, "A Natural Approach to Bone Health," informational letter to health professionals, 1998.

15. Bodmer, "Women's Health News: The Latest Healing Breakthroughs for Women," 4. Reporting on a study by gynecologist Dr. Guy Abraham.

16. Summarized from Gero Vita Laboratories product information guide.

17. Gaby, *Preventing and Reversing Osteoporosis,* 42.

18. Ibid.

19. Ibid., 101.

20. Jackson and Teague, *The Handbook of Alternatives to Chemical Medicine,* 144.

21. *Standard Process Clinical Reference Guide,* 30.

22. *The Training Session: Introduction to Standard Process,* 12.

23. *Standard Process Clinical Reference Guide,* 8–9.

24. Colgan, *Hormonal Health,* 229.

25. William Campbell Douglass, M.D., "Astonishing New Cure Reverses Osteoporosis," *Health Breakthroughs* (winter 1997): 12.

26. Ibid.

27. Isadore Rosenfeld, M.D., *Dr. Rosenfeld's Guide to Alternative Medicine* (New York: Random House, 1996), 317.

28. Gaby, *Preventing and Reversing Osteoporosis,* 82.

29. Nancy Appleton, Ph.D., *Healthy Bones: What You Should Know about Osteoporosis* (Garden City Park, NY: Avery, 1991).

30. Jackson and Teague, *The Handbook of Alternatives to Chemical Medicine,* 147.

31. Gaby, *Preventing and Reversing Osteoporosis,* 93.

32. Ibid., 18.

33. Ibid., 94; Jackson and Teague, *The Handbook of Alternatives to Chemical Medicine,* 145.

34. Gaby, *Preventing and Reversing Osteoporosis,* 85–86.

35. Ibid., 97.

36. Glenn Miller, M.D., "What Are Some Benefits from Exposure to Sunlight?" *Ukiah Daily Journal* (March 19, 1998): 3.

37. Ralph W. Moss, Ph.D., "New Evidence on Old Vitamin: Vitamin D May Combat Breast, Colon and Prostate Cancer," *The Cancer Chronicles,* no. 32–33 (June 1996). Available at www.ralphmoss.com/vitaminD.html.

38. *Taber's Cyclopedic Medical Dictionary,* v–23.

39. Hector DeLuca, "The Real 'Good News' for Osteoporosis Sufferers," *Bio/Tech News:* 4.

40. Bruce West, D.C., "Butter and Booze," *Health Alert,* vol. 15, no. 9 (September 1998): 1–2.

41. G. C. Supplee, S. Ansbacher, R. Bender, and G. Flinigan, "The Influence of Milk Constituents on the Effectiveness of Vitamin D," *Journal of Biological Chemistry,* 141 (May 1936): 95–107.

42. Balch and Balch, *Prescription for Nutritional Healing,* 20.

43. Gaby, *Preventing and Reversing Osteoporosis,* 22–23.

44. Balch and Balch, *Prescription for Nutritional Healing,* 20; Brown, *Better Bones, Better Body,* 394; *Taber's Cyclopedic Medical Dictionary,* v–24.

45. Balch and Balch, *Prescription for Nutritional Healing,* 20.

46. Available at www.merck.com/pubs/mmanual/section1/chapter3/3i.htm.

47. Dobbins, "Effective Nutrition Therapy."

48. LeRoy, "Major Study Results Challenge Claims for Dairy," 18.

49. *Standard Process Clinical Reference Guide,* 29.

50. Balch and Balch, *Prescription for Nutritional Healing,* 414.

51. Consumer Reports Books, *The New Medicine Show: Consumers Union's New Practical Guide to Some Everyday Health Products* (Mount Vernon, NY: Consumer Reports Books, 1989), 204.

52. Ibid., 206.

53. *Standard Process Clinical Reference Guide,* 9.

54. Versendaal, author's interview.

55. Newell, author's interview.

56. Donald Warren, D.D.S., author's interview.

57. Versendaal, author's interview.

58. Newell, author's interview; *Standard Process Clinical Reference Guide,* 10.

59. Dobbins, "Effective Nutrition Therapy."

60. Ibid.

Chapter 8

1. Dobbins, "Effective Nutrition Therapy."

2. *Taber's Cyclopedic Medical Dictionary,* 31.

3. *20/20,* ABC network, April 10, 1998.

4. Balch and Balch, *Prescription for Nutritional Healing,* 51.

5. Ibid., 51.

6. *Taber's Cyclopedic Medical Dictionary,* 59.

7. Bodmer with Fuchs, *Stop Breast Cancer before It Happens,* 7.

8. Hunter Yost, M.D., "Molecules for the Mind," *Arizona Star* (no date).

9. International Hemp Association, "Hemp as an Industrial and Food Source," available at http://mojo.calyx.net/~olsen/HEMP/hemptoc.html.

10. Dobbins, "Effective Nutrition Therapy."

11. Mack, author's interview.

12. Dobbins, "Effective Nutrition Therapy."

13. Anne Louise Gittleman, M.S., *Beyond Pritikin* (New York: Bantam, 1989). Quoted in Jade Beutler, R.R.T., R.C.P., "Weight Loss with Flax Seed Oil: The Non-Fat Fat," *Health Perspectives,* available at www.barleans.com/literature/61-weightloss.pdf.

14. *Standard Process Clinical Reference Guide,* 15.

15. Dobbins, "Effective Nutrition Therapy."

16. Mary Frost, M.A., *Going Back to the Basics of Human Health: Avoiding the Fads, the Trends and the Bold-Faced Lies,* self-published, February 1997, 28.

17. Yost, "Molecules for the Mind."

18. Dobbins, "Effective Nutrition Therapy."

19. Ibid.

20. Balch and Balch, *Prescription for Nutritional Healing,* 51.

21. Dobbins, "Effective Nutrition Therapy."

22. Available at www.cspinet.org/olestra.

23. Dobbins, "Effective Nutrition Therapy."

24. Royal Lee, *Therapeutic Food Manual.*

25. Frost, *Going Back to the Basics of Human Health*, 28.

26. Yost, "Molecules for the Mind."

27. Donald Rudin, M.D., and Clara Felix, *Omega-3 Oils* (Garden City Park, NY: Avery, 1996), 7.

28. Whole Health Discount Center, "Essential Fatty Acids," available at www.health-pages.com/fa.

29. *Standard Process Clinical Reference Guide,* 2.

30. Ibid.

31. Dobbins, "Effective Nutrition Therapy."

32. Ibid.

33. *Standard Process Clinical Reference Guide,* 7.

34. Newell, author's interview.

35. Bruce West, D.C., "Kidney Stone Facts," *Health Alert,* vol. 15, no. 7 (July 1998): 4.

36. Ibid.

37. N. Claassen, et al., "The Effect of Different n-6/n-3 Essential Fatty Acid Ratios on Calcium Balance and Bone in Rats," *Prostaglandins Leukot Essent Fatty Acids,* 53 (1995): 13–19.

38. N. Claassen, et al., "Supplemented Gamma-Linolenic Acid and Eicosapentaenoic Acid Influence Bone Status in Young Male Rats: Effects on Free Urinary Collagen Crosslinks, Total Urinary Hydroxyproline, and Bone Calcium Content," *Bone,* 16 (1995): 385S–392S.

39. *Standard Process Clinical Reference Guide,* 25.

40. Ibid., 15.

41. *Standard Process Clinical Reference Guide,* 33.

42. Dobbins, "Effective Nutrition Therapy"; letter from Royal Lee, D.D.S., private collection, July 21, 1948.

43. D. A. Versendaal, D.C., Ph.D., and Dawn Versendaal-Hoezee, *Contact Reflex Analysis and Designed Clinical Nutrition: A Healing Art* (Holland, MI: Hoezee Marketing, 1997), 116.

Chapter 9

1. Newell, author's interview.

2. Bruce West, D.C., author's interview, summer 1998.

3. Ibid., 32.

4. Gaby, *Preventing and Reversing Osteoporosis,* 231.

5. Newell, author's interview.

6. *Standard Process Clinical Reference Guide,* 10.

7. Brown, *Better Bones, Better Body,* 183.

8. Ibid., 183–84.

9. Henry R. Harrower, M.D., *Practical Endocrinology,* 2nd edition (Milwaukee, WI: Lee Foundation for Nutritional Research, 1957), 46.

10. John Lee, *Natural Progesterone,* 53.

11. Ibid., 55.

12. J. C. Prior. "Progesterone As a Bone-Trophic Hormone," *Endocrine Reviews,* vol. 11, no. 2 (May 1990), 386.

13. John Lee, *Natural Progesterone,* 69.

14. John Lee, M.D., with Virginia Hopkins, *What Your Doctor May Not Tell You about Menopause: The Breakthrough Book on Natural Progesterone* (New York: Warner, 1996), 79.

15. I. R. Reid, et al., "Testosterone Therapy in Glucocorticoid-Treated Men," *Archives of Internal Medicine,* vol. 156, no. 11 (June 1996): 1173–77.

16. Brown, *Better Bones, Better Body,* 188.

17. Jim Paterson, "Is There 'Male Menopause'?" *USA Weekend* (January 2–4, 1998): 16.

18. John Lee with Hopkins, *What Your Doctor May Not Tell You about Menopause,* xvii.

19. Kerri Bodmer, "Health Secrets for Women Only," *Women's Health Letter,* supplement (October 1998): 7.

20. Dover, *Osteoporosis.*

21. Brown, *Better Bones, Better Body,* 188.

22. John Lee with Hopkins, *What Your Doctor May Not Tell You about Menopause,* 128.

23. Paterson, "Is There 'Male Menopause'?" 16.

24. Ego Seeman, M.D., "Osteoporosis in Men," presented at the Twenty-

Third Annual Meeting of the American Society of Bone Mineral Research, October 2001.

25. Harrower, *Practical Endocrinology,* 133.

26. Dobbins, "Effective Nutrition Therapy."

27. John Lee with Hopkins, *What Your Doctor May* Not *Tell You about Menopause,* 110.

28. Baylor College of Medicine, "Daughters of Women Exposed to DES Have No Increased Cancer Risk" (1998), available at http://public.bcm.tmc.edu:80/pa/descancerrisk.htm.

29. Maureen Schaub, author's interview.

30. Amanda McQuade Crawford, M.N.I.M.H., *Herbal Remedies for Women: Discover Nature's Wonderful Secrets Just for Women* (Rocklin, CA: Prima Publishing, 1997), 12–13

31. *Standard Process Clinical Reference Guide,* 21.

32. "Symptom Survey Form," *Standard Process Clinical Reference Guide,* 4.

33. Versendaal, author's interview.

34. Gaby, *Preventing and Reversing Osteoporosis,* 163–65.

35. Bruce West, D.C., "DHEA and Insulin: The Facts," *Health Alert,* vol. 15, no. 2 (February 1998): 4.

36. Bruce West, D.C., "More on DHEA" *Health Alert,* vol 14, no. 7 (July 1997): 3.

37. Dobbins, "Effective Nutrition Therapy."

38. Ibid.

39. *Standard Process Clinical Reference Guide,* 2.

40. *The Training Session: Introduction to Standard Process,* 17; see also "Symptom Survey Form," *Standard Process Clinical Reference Guide,* 4.

41. Crawford, *Herbal Remedies for Women,* 5.

42. Mack, author's interview.

43. *Standard Process Clinical Reference Guide,* 28.

44. Ibid., 30.

45. Ibid., 31.

46. Versendaal and Versendaal-Hoezee, *Contact Reflex Analysis and Designed Clinical Nutrition,* 46.

47. Mack, author's interview.

48. Debbie Moskowitz, N.D., "Phytoestrogens: An Exciting Alternative," reprinted from *Natural Solutions,* vol. 4, no. 4 (fall 1996). Available at http://womenatmidlife.com/headlines/phytoestrogens.htm.

49. "Menopause," *Transitions for Women* (fall 1997/winter 1998): 3.

50. Douglass, "Say Goodbye to Illness," 12.

51. John Lee with Hopkins, *What Your Doctor May* Not *Tell You about Menopause,* 78.

52. Ibid., 35.

53. Ibid., 47.

54. Newell, author's interview.

55. Mack, author's interview.

Chapter 10

1. National Institutes of Health, Office of the Director, *NIH Consensus Statement*, vol. 12, no. 4 (June 6–8, 1994): 14.

2. Doug Hullander and Patrick L. Barry, "Space Bones," *Science at NASA* (October 1, 1999), available at http://science.nasa.gov/headlines/y2001/ast01oct_1.htm.

3. Dover, *Osteoporosis*, 18.

4. Ibid., 18.

5. "Calcium: Beneficial to Bones and More," 17.

6. Osteoporosis Prevention Project, *Osteoporosis and You* (Denver, CO: Department of Health), vol. 1, no. 3.

7. Claire Martin, "Prescriptions: A Positive Impact," *Outside* (December 1997), available at http://web.outsideonline.com/magazine/1297/9712bodypre.html.

8. Christina Brown, available at www.indianropemassage.com/Publications.htm.

9. Julie Jacobs, personal communication.

10. Janet Raloff, "Medicinal EMFs: Harnessing Electric and Magnetic Fields for Healing and Health," *Science News Online* (November 13, 1999), available at www.sciencenews.org/sn_arc99/11_13_99/bob2.htm.

11. Jane Barton Hamilton, Ph.D., R.D., C.N.S, Magnetico Sleep Pads advertisment.

12. Dover, *Osteoporosis*, 16.

13. Claire Martin, "A Positive Impact," *Outside* (December 1997): 150.

14. Sharon Bortz, "Calcium: Part Three," *Redwood Health Club Newsletter* (November 1997): 1.

15. E. J. Bendavid, J. Shan, and E. Barrett-Conner, "Factors Associated with Bone Mineral Density in Middle-Aged Men," *Journal of Bone Mineral Research*, vol. 11, no. 8 (August 1996): 1185–90.

16. Available at www.orthohelp.com/osteoprx.htm.

17. Gaby, *Preventing and Reversing Osteoporosis*, 147.

18. Mack, author's interview.

19. West, author's interview.

20. Dobbins, "Effective Nutrition Therapy."

21. William Eicher, editor, *American Council on Collaborative Medicine*, vol. 4, no. 5 (May 1998): 2.

22. Mack, author's interview.

23. Dobbins, "Effective Nutrition Therapy."

24. Ibid.

25. Fred Ulan, D.C., C.C.N., "Preventing Recurring Subluxations with CRA," *The American Chiropractor* (September/October 1998): 26–40.

26. Dobbins, "Effective Nutrition Therapy."

27. D'Adamo, *4 Your Type* catalog, 24.

28. Dobbins, "Effective Nutrition Therapy."

29. Ibid.

Chapter 11

1. Mack, author's interview.

2. George Higashida, President of Sun Wellness. Letter to Health-Conscious Friends, undated.

3. Hollie Shaner, M.S.A., R.N., "Five Minutes with Hollie Shaner," *NurseWeek* (April 19, 1999): 8.

4. Brenda Biondo, "Are Common Chemicals Scrambling Your Hormones?" *USA Weekend* (February 13–15, 1998): 18.

5. Gaby, *Preventing and Reversing Osteoporosis*, 16.

6. Mack, author's interview.

7. Ibid.

8. LeRoy, "Major Study Results Challenge Claims for Dairy," 18–19.

9. Ibid.

10. National Institutes of Health, *NIH Consensus Statement*, 15.

11. Versendaal and Versendaal-Hoezee, *Contact Reflex Analysis and Designed Clinical Nutrition*, 39.

12. Gaby, *Preventing and Reversing Osteoporosis*, 11.

13. Royal Lee, talk for the American Academy of Nutrition Society.

14. Jean Carper, "Eat Smart," *USA Weekend* (November 6–8, 1998): 15.

15. Bruce West, D.C., "Diabetes, Corn Syrup, and Chlorine," *Health Alert*, vol. 15, no. 7 (July 1998): 6.

16. Mack, author's interview.

17. Dobbins, "Effective Nutrition Therapy."

18. Ibid.

19. Grocery Manufacturers of America, available at www.gmabrands.com/facts/biotechnology.cfm.

20. Judith DeCava, M.S., C.C.N. "Let Food Be Your Medicine," *Nutrition News* (March/April 2002): 1.

21. Newell, author's interview.

22. John Lee, *Natural Progesterone*, 81–82.

23. Dobbins, "Effective Nutrition Therapy."

24. Bruce West, D.C., "How Many Prescriptions?" *Health Alert*, vol. 15, no. 4 (April 1998): 5.

25. National Institutes of Health, *NIH Consensus Statement*, 14–15.

26. Brown, *Better Bones, Better Body*, 165–66.

27. Gaby, *Preventing and Reversing Osteoporosis*, 206.

28. Ibid., 208.

29. Ibid., 211.

30. Megan Flaherty, "Healthy Planet: Hospitals Learn to Clean Up Their Act," *NurseWeek*, vol. 12, no. 2 (January 25, 1999): 1.

31. Warren, author's interview.

32. Reported in "Price-Pottenger Foundation Newsletter," *Acupuncture and Electro-Therapeutics*, 20 (1995): 133–48.

33. Dobbins, "Effective Nutrition Therapy."

34. Ibid.

35. Royal Lee, talk for the American Academy of Nutrition Society.

36. John Yiamouyiannis, Ph.D., "Lifesavers Guide to Fluoridation, Risks/Benefits Evaluated" (Delaware, OH: Safe Water Foundation, 1988), 1–6.

37. Michael Smatt, D.C., "Gloria Steinem," *Today's Chiropractic* (March/April 1996): 76–80.

38. D. A. Versendaal, D.C., Ph.D., seminar, Oakland, CA, January 1998.

39. Mack, author's interview.

40. Ibid.

41. Dobbins, "Effective Nutrition Therapy."

42. Fred Ulan, D.C., C.C.N., "Autonomic Response Testing," seminar, Berkeley, CA, January 2002.

43. Versendaal and Versendaal-Hoezee, *Contact Reflex Analysis and Designed Clinical Nutrition*, 140.

44. Dobbins, "Effective Nutrition Therapy."

45. Ibid.

46. *The Training Session: Introduction to Standard Process*, 34.

47. Dobbins, "Effective Nutrition Therapy."

48. Ibid.

49. Ibid.

50. Versendaal and Versendaal-Hoezee, *Contact Reflex Analysis and Designed Clinical Nutrition*, 26.

51. David N. Holvey, M.D., editor, *The Merck Manual*, 12th edition, (Rathway, NJ: Merck and Co., 1972), 15.

52. D'Adamo, *4 Your Type* catalog, 13.

53. Crawford, *Herbal Remedies for Women*, 5.

PART THREE

Chapter 12

1. Newell, author's interview.

Chapter 13

1. Mack, author's interview.
2. Dobbins, "Effective Nutrition Therapy."

Chapter 14

1. Dobbins, "Effective Nutrition Therapy."
2. Royal Lee, *Therapeutic Food Manual*, 219.
3. Dobbins, "Effective Nutrition Therapy."
4. Mack, author's interview.
5. Versendaal, author's interview.
6. Mack, author's interview.
7. Versendaal and Versendaal-Hoezee, *Contact Reflex Analysis and Designed Clinical Nutrition*.
8. West, author's interview, January 1999.
9. Dobbins, "Effective Nutrition Therapy."
10. Royal Lee, *Therapeutic Food Manual*, 219.

Chapter 15

1. West, author's interview, summer 1998.
2. Ibid.
3. Price, *Nutrition and Physical Degeneration*.

BIBLIOGRAPHY

Abraham, G. E., and Grewal, H. "A Total Dietary Program Emphasizing Magnesium Instead of Calcium: Effect on the Mineral Density of Cacaneous Bone in Postmenopausal Women on Hormonal Therapy." *Journal of Reproductive Medicine,* vol. 35, no. 5, May 1990.

American Council on Collaborative Medicine, vol. 4, no. 5, May 1998.

Appleton, Nancy. *Healthy Bones: What You Should Know about Osteoporosis.* Garden City Park, NY: Avery, 1991.

Atkins, Robert C., M.D. *Dr. Atkins' New Diet Revolution.* New York: Avon Health, 1997.

Balch, James, M.D., and Phyllis A. Balch, C.N.C. *Prescription for Nutritional Healing,* 2nd edition. Garden City Park, NY: Avery, 1997.

Barilla, Jean, M.S. "Rx for Health Care." *The Physicians Newsletter: Health through Nutrition,* vol. 2, no. 1, April 1997.

Baurac, Deborah. "Joint Exchange." *Modern Maturity,* September/October 1997.

Bendavid, E. J., J. Shan, and E. Barrett-Conner. "Factors Associated with Bone Mineral Density in Middle-Aged Men." *Journal of Bone Mineral Research,* vol. 11, no. 8, August 1996.

Biondo, Brenda. "Are Common Chemicals Scrambling Your Hormones?" *USA Weekend,* February 13–15, 1998.

Black, Dean. "Artful Science: Documenting the Chiropractic Experience." Parker College (unpublished article), 1996. Quoted in Peter Clecak, Ph.D., "Giving Patients 'Reasonable Counsel': The Case of Contact Reflex Analysis." *Alternative Medicine Journal,* July/August 1994.

Bodmer, Kerri. "Don't Let New Fosamax Study Fool You." *Women's Health Letter,* vol. 7, no. 4, April 1998.

———. "Editronate and Osteoporosis." *Women's Health Letter,* vol. 7, no. 5, May 1998.

————. *Got Milk? Get Heart Disease.* Atlanta, GA: Soundview Publications, Inc., 1996.

————. "Health Secrets for Women Only." *Women's Health Letter,* supplement, October 1998.

————. "Healthy Body, Healthy Bones." *Women's Health Letter,* vol. 6, no. 7, July 1998.

————. *Osteoporosis and the Calcium Controversy.* Atlanta, GA: Soundview Publications, Inc., 1996.

————. "Update on Calcium Channel Blockers." *Women's Health Letter,* vol. 7, no. 5, May 1998.

————, with Nan Kathryn Fuchs. *Stop Breast Cancer before It Happens.* Atlanta, GA: Soundview Publications, Inc., 1997.

Bone, Kerry. *Clinical Applications of Ayurvedic and Chinese Herbs: Monographs for the Western Herbal Practitioner.* Queensland, Australia: Phytotherapy Press, 1996.

Bortz, Sharon, R.D. "Boning Up on Calcium." *Redwood Health Club Newsletter,* September 1997.

————. "Calcium: Part Three." *Redwood Health Club Newsletter,* November 1997.

Brown, Susan E., Ph.D. *Better Bones, Better Body.* New Canaan, CT: Keats Publishing Company, 1996.

"Calcium: Beneficial to Bones and More." *Healthy Cell News,* spring/summer 1996.

Carper, Jean. "Calcium: Not for Women Only." *USA Weekend,* March 27–29, 1999.

Center for Science in the Public Interest. "P&G, Frito-Lay, Set to Unleash Diarrhea-Causing Olestra on Americans," *What's New,* February 5, 1998. Available at www.cspinet.org/olestra.

Clecak, Peter, Ph.D., Ron Carsten, D.V.M., M.S., Paul Jasoviak, D.C., Mary Jane Mack, R.N., Steve Nelson, Phar.D., Ph.D., Michael Robertson, M.D., J. Rodney Shelley, D.C., and Donald Warren, D.D.S., F.A.H.N.P. "Alternative Healing Modes: A Look at Contact Reflex Analysis." *Alternative Medicine Journal,* July/August 1994.

Colgan, Michael. *Hormonal Health: Nutritional and Hormonal Strategies for Emotional Well-Being and Intellectual Longevity.* Vancouver, British Columbia, Canada: Apple Publishing, 1996.

The Complete Book of Natural and Medicinal Cures: How to Choose the Most Potent Healing Agents for over 300 Conditions and Diseases. Edited by *Prevention Magazine* Health Books. Emmaus, PA: Rodale Press, 1994.

Consumer Reports Books. *The New Medicine Show: Consumers Union's New Practical Guide to Some Everyday Health Products.* Mount Vernon, NY, 1989.

Corces, Arturo, M.D. Summarized remarks at conferences of the National Institutes of Health Osteoporosis and Related Bone Diseases National Resource Center, National Osteoporosis Foundation. Washington, DC: National Institutes of Health, June 1996 and July 1997.

Courtney, John, and Royal Lee. *Conversations in Nutrition.* Unpublished notes from question and answer sessions with health professionals.

Crawford, Amanda McQuade, M.N.I.M.H. *The Herbal Menopause Book: Herbs, Nutrition and Other Natural Therapies.* Freedom, CA: Crossing Press, 1996.

———. *Herbal Remedies for Women: Discover Nature's Wonderful Secrets Just for Women.* Rocklin, CA: Prima Publishing, 1977.

D'Adamo, Peter, N.D. *Eat Right for Your Type.* New York: Riverhead/Putnam, 1996.

DeCava, Judith A., M.S., C.C.N. *The Real Truth about Vitamins and Antioxidants.* Columbus, GA: Brentwood Academic Press, 1996.

Deets, Horace B. "AARP's Realignment." AARP Perspectives, *Modern Maturity,* November/December 1997.

Douglass, William Campbell, M.D. "Astonishing New Cure Reverses Osteoporosis." *Health Breakthroughs,* winter 1997.

———. "Say Goodbye to Illness." *Health Breakthroughs,* fall 1997.

———. "Steps toward Beating Osteoporosis." *Second Opinion,* November 1995.

Dover, Clare. *Osteoporosis.* London, England: Ward Lock in conjunction with the National Osteoporosis Society, 1994.

Dufty, William. *Sugar Blues.* New York: Warner Books, 1975.

Eades, Michael R., M.D., and Mary Dan Eades, M.D. *Protein Power.* New York: Bantam, 1998.

Flaherty, Megan. "Healthy Planet: Hospitals Learn to Clean Up Their Act." *NurseWeek,* vol. 12, no. 2, January 25, 1999.

Frost, Mary, M.A. *Going Back to the Basics of Human Health: Avoiding the Fads, the Trends and the Bold-Faced Lies.* Self-published, February 1997.

Fuchs, Nan Kathryn, Ph.D. "The Nutrition Detective." *Women's Health Letter,* vol. 7, no. 4, April 1998.

Gaby, Alan, M.D. *Preventing and Reversing Osteoporosis: Every Woman's Essential Guide.* Rocklin, CA: Prima Publishing, 1994.

Gittleman, Ann Louise, M.S. *Beyond Pritikin.* New York: Bantam Books, 1989.

Green, Jerry, J.D. "Collaborative Physician-Patient Planning and Professional Liability: Opening the Legal Door to Unconventional Medicine." *Advances in Mind-Body Medicine,* vol. 15, no. 2, spring 1999.

———. "The Health Care Contract: A Model for Sharing Responsibility." *Somatics,* vol. 3, no. 4, 1982.

Griggs, Barbara. *Green Pharmacy.* Rochester, VT: Healing Arts Press, 1997.

Harrower, Henry R., M.D. *Practical Endocrinology,* 2nd edition. Milwaukee, WI: Lee Foundation for Nutritional Research, 1957.

Hellinghausen, Mary Ann, Leigh Morgan, and Valeria J. Nelson. *NurseWeek,* June 23, 1997.

Hemp Food Industries Association. "Hemp Seed Nutrition: A Perfect Balance." Available at www.hemp.co.uk/html/nutinfo.html.

Hermann, Mindy. "A Call for Calcium." *Modern Maturity,* March/April 1998.

Higashida, George. Letter to Health-Conscious Friends. Sun Wellness, Inc. (no date).

Jackson, Donna M. *The Bone Detectives: How Forensic Anthropologists Solve Crimes and Uncover Mysteries of the Dead.* Boston: Little, Brown, & Co., 1996.

Jackson, Mildred, N.D., and Terri Teague. *The Handbook of Alternatives to Chemical Medicine.* Oakland, CA: self-published, 1975.

Jensen, Bernard, and Mark Anderson. *Empty Harvest: Understanding the Link between Our Food, Our Immunity, and Our Planet.* Garden City Park, NY: Avery, 1990.

Journal of the American Dietetic Association, March 1995. Available at www.eatright.com/images/journal/0101/adap0101.pdf.

Lanucci, Lisa. "Bone Power." *Energy Times,* May 1997.

Lee, John, M.D. *Natural Progesterone: The Multiple Roles of a Remarkable Hormone.* Sebastopol, CA: BLL Publishing, 1993.

———. "Osteoporosis Reversal: The Role of Progesterone." *The International Clinical Nutrition Review,* vol. 10, no. 3, July 1990.

———, with Virginia Hopkins. *What Your Doctor May Not Tell You about Menopause: The Breakthrough Book on Natural Progesterone.* New York: Warner, 1996.

Lee, Royal, D.D.S. "Food Integrity." *Conversations in Nutrition,* April 1955.

———. *The Principles of Cell Auto-Regulation.* 1947.

———. *Therapeutic Food Manual.* Publication date unknown.

LeRoy, Bob, R.D. "Major Study Results Challenge Claims for Dairy." *Vegetarian Voice,* fall 1997.

Malka, Jeffrey, S.M. "Treatment of Osteoporosis Today." Available at www.orthohelp.com/osteoprx.htm.

Martin, Claire. "A Positive Impact." *Outside,* December 1997.

Miller, Glenn, M.D. "What Are Some Benefits from Exposure to Sunlight?" *Ukiah Daily Journal,* March 19, 1998.

Mills, Simon, and Kerry Bone. *Principles and Practice of Phytotherapy: Modern Herbal Medicine.* Edinburgh, Scotland: Churchill Livingstone, 2000.

MPI NuPro. "Natural vs. Synthetic (Is Natural Better?)." *The NuPro Therapist,* vol. 2, no. 2.

Murray, Michael, N.D. "The *True* Arthritis Cure." In *Arthritis Counselor,* special edition, 1997.

National Osteoporosis Foundation. "Men with Osteoporosis, in Their Own Words." Washington DC: National Osteoporosis Foundation, 1997.

National Institutes of Health, Office of the Director. "Optimal Calcium Intake." *NIH Consensus Statement,* vol. 12, no. 4, June 6–8, 1994.

Northrup, Christiane, M.D. *Women's Bodies, Women's Wisdom: Creating Physical and Emotional Health and Healing.* New York: Bantam, 1998.

Osteoporosis and You. Denver, CO: Colorado Department of Health, Osteoporosis Prevention Project, vol. 1, no. 3.

Paterson, Jim. "Is There 'Male Menopause'?" *USA Weekend,* January 2–4, 1998.

Percival, Mark. "Bone Health and Osteoporosis." *Clinical Nutrition Insights,* vol. 5, no. 4, 1998.

Price, Westin. *Nutrition and Physical Degeneration.* La Mesa, CA: Price-Pottenger Nutritional Foundation, 1939.

"Price-Pottenger Foundation Newsletter." *Acupuncture and Electro-Therapeutics,* 20, 1995.

Prior, J. C. "Progesterone As a Bone-Trophic Hormone." *Endocrine Reviews,* vol. 11, no. 2, May 1990.

Quillman, Susan M., R.N., M.N. *Nutrition and Diet Therapy,* 2nd edition. Springhouse, PA: Springhouse Notes, 1994.

Reid, I. R., and others. "Testosterone Therapy in Glucocorticoid-Treated Men." *Archives of Internal Medicine,* no. 11, June 1996.

Robbins, John. *Reclaiming Our Health: Exploding the Medical Myth and Embracing the Source of True Healing.* Tiburon, CA: H. J. Kramer, 1996.

Rosenfeld, Isadore, M.D. *Dr. Rosenfeld's Guide to Alternative Medicine.* New York: Random House, 1996.

Schmidt, D. Raymond. "A Treatment for Leprosy." *Health Journal,* Price-Pottenger Nutrition Foundation, vol. 21, no. 3, fall 1997.

Shaner, Hollie, M.S.A., R.N. Interview, "Five Minutes with Hollie Shaner." *NurseWeek,* April 19, 1999.

Sheehy, Gail. *New Passages: Mapping Your Life across Time.* New York: Random House, 1995.

Shefi, Ron. "Contact Reflex Analysis." *CRA Collector's Edition.*

Simons, Wallace, R.Ph. "A Pharmacist Explores Some Differences between Natural Progesterone and Synthetic Progestins." *Women's Health Connections,* no. 2b, 1997.

Smatt, Michael. "Gloria Steinem." *Today's Chiropractic,* March/April 1996.

"Sulfur: An Ancient Nutrient Needed Now, More Than Ever Before." *American Council on Collaborative Medicine,* vol. 4, no. 3, March 1998.

Supplee, G. C., S. Ansbacher, R. Bender, and G. Flinigan. "The Influence of Milk Constiuents on the Effectiveness of Vitamin D." *Journal of Biological Chemistry,* 141, May 1936.

Taber's Cyclopedic Medical Dictionary, 8th edition. Philadelphia, PA: F. A. David Company, 1960.

Theodosakis, Jason, M.D., M.S., M.P.H., Brenda Adderly, M.H.A., and Barry Fox, Ph.D. *The Arthritis Cure.* New York: St. Martin's Press, 1997.

Therapeutic Food Manual. An unpublished compilation of nutritional information gathered from health care practitioners.

Ulan, Fred, D.C., C.C.N. "Preventing Recurring Subluxations with CRA." *The American Chiropractor,* September/October 1998.

Versendaal, D.C., Ph.D., and Dawn Versendaal-Hoezee. *Contact Reflex Analysis and Designed Clinical Nutrition: A Healing Art.* Holland, MI: Hoezee Marketing, 1993.

Versendaal, D.C., Ph.D. "CRA Technology and Osteoporosis: The 'Brittle Bone' Syndrome." *Contact Reflex Analysis Seminar Papers* (distributed seminar packet), Oakland, CA, summer 1998.

Wardlaw, Gordon M. "Putting Body Weight and Osteoporosis into Perspective," *American Journal of Clinical Nutrition,* supplement 433-6S, March 1996.

West, Bruce. "Butter and Booze." *Health Alert,* vol. 15, no. 9, July 1998.

———. "DHEA and Insulin: The Facts." *Health Alert,* vol. 15, no. 2, February 1998.

———. "Diabetes, Corn Syrup, and Chlorine." *Health Alert,* vol. 15, no. 7, July 1998.

———. "Diseases of Calcium Metabolism." *Health Alert,* vol. 15, no. 5, May 1998.

———. "High Dose Vitamin C Causes Problems." *Health Alert,* vol. 15, no. 9, July 1998.

———. "How Many Prescriptions?" *Health Alert,* vol. 15, no. 4, April 1998.

———. "Kidney Diseases, Blood Pressure and Glaucoma." *Health Alert,* vol. 14, no. 7, July 1997.

———. "Kidney Stone Facts." *Health Alert,* vol. 15, no. 7, July 1998.

———. "More on DHEA." *Health Alert,* vol. 14, no. 7, July 1997.

Whitaker, Julian, M.D. "Health Breakthroughs." *Second Opinion,* spring 1998.

Wyeth-Ayerst Laboratories advertisement, *USA Weekend Magazine,* September 26–28, 1997.

Yiamouyiannis, John, Ph.D. *Lifesavers Guide to Fluoridation: Risks/Benefits Evaluated.* Delaware, OH: Safe Water Foundation, 1988.

Yost, Hunter, M.D. "Molecules for the Mind." *The Arizona Daily Star,* no date.

INDEX

ABOUT THE AUTHOR

PAMELA LEVIN, R.N., is an award-winning author and nutritional journalist who draws on thirty years of experience in the health field. After recovering her own bone health, she compiled *Perfect Bones* out of gratitude for the methods described in these pages.

Pamela is a graduate of the University of Illinois College of Nursing, Chicago, and has over 150 hours of postgraduate education in advanced clinical nutrition. She studied transactional analysis with its founder, Eric Berne, and became the first nurse to be awarded clinical and teaching membership in its international organization. She has taught and trained health professionals in fifty-one U.S. cities and in six foreign countries on four different continents.

Her other writings, now in ten languages, include numerous published articles and four books that have sold over one hundred thousand copies worldwide. Pamela is founder and publisher of the Nourishing Company, which published the first edition of *Perfect Bones.* She has been in private practice since 1970 and is the mother of two grown children.